Reconnecting after Isolation

A Johns Hopkins Press Health Book

RECONNECTING

after ISOLATION

Coping with Anxiety, Depression, Grief, PTSD, and More

Susan J. Noonan, MD, MPH

JOHNS HOPKINS UNIVERSITY PRESS
Baltimore

Note to the reader: This book is not meant to substitute for medical care of people who have depression or other mental disorders, and treatment should not be based solely on its contents. Instead, treatment must be developed in a dialogue between the individual and their physician. My book has been written to help with that dialogue.

© 2022 Johns Hopkins University Press
All rights reserved. Published 2022
Printed in the United States of America on acid-free paper
9 8 7 6 5 4 3 2 1

Johns Hopkins University Press
2715 North Charles Street
Baltimore, Maryland 21218-4363
www.press.jhu.edu

Library of Congress Cataloging-in-Publication Data

Names: Noonan, Susan J., 1953– author.
Title: Reconnecting after isolation : coping with anxiety, depression,
  grief, PTSD, and more / Susan J. Noonan, MD, MPH.
Description: Baltimore : Johns Hopkins University Press, [2022]
  | Series: A Johns Hopkins Press health book | Includes
  bibliographical references and index.
Identifiers: LCCN 2021046919 | ISBN 9781421444222 (hardcover ; alk.
  paper) | ISBN 9781421444239 (paperback ; alk. paper) |
  ISBN 9781421444246 (ebook)
Subjects: LCSH: Social isolation—Psychological aspects. | Loneliness.
  | Interpersonal relations. | Social interaction.
Classification: LCC BF575.L7 N66 2022 | DDC 302.5/45—dc23
LC record available at https://lccn.loc.gov/2021046919

A catalog record for this book is available from the British Library.

*Special discounts are available for bulk purchases of this book. For more
information, please contact Special Sales at specialsales@jh.edu.*

"A [mental] health charity called the Bearded Fishermen has begun a nightly suicide-prevention patrol in and around Gainsborough, [England,] . . . looking for people in crisis due to the coronavirus pandemic." Founded by two men who have firsthand experience with depression, anxiety, and suicide attempts, they are part of Night Watch, an initiative to monitor known suicide hot spots in the area, working with emergency responders and the community. There has been a measurable increase in calls for support and their crisis services as the community struggles through the coronavirus pandemic.

"The situation in the Gainsborough area reflects the larger mental health strain across Britain [and the world] . . . Research has shown a rise in reports of loneliness, a particular concern for young people, difficulties for those with pre-existing mental health issues and an increase in reports of suicidal ideation. The impact of the pandemic and its effect—lockdowns, an economic downturn and social isolation—on mental health . . . could be felt for years to come."

Megan Specia, *New York Times*,
December 6, 2020

Contents

Acknowledgments

I was greatly honored when asked to write this book on the mental health consequences of social isolation using our collective experience of the COVID-19 pandemic as an example. Digging down deep and writing about such a sensitive topic would not have been possible without the support of those in my life who keep me afloat. I continue to owe limitless thanks and appreciation to Drs. Andrew Nierenberg, Jonathan Alpert, and Timothy Petersen and to the close friends and family who have sustained me throughout.

No book is published alone. I want to acknowledge the openness, perception, and unique contributions of Drs. Thea Gallagher, Wendy Silverman, Douglas Katz, and Sheila Rauch—their real-time clinical input has greatly enhanced this manuscript.

Most important, the insightful staff of Johns Hopkins University Press have rightfully earned my profound gratitude and praise, including Joe Rusko, Juliana McCarthy, Melanie Mallon, and others. They guided me in addressing this topic in a uniquely perceptive, meticulous, and thoughtful manner.

Reconnecting after Isolation

Introduction

We've all been there at one time or another—caught in the sense of being alone and far apart from others, leaving us feeling lost, anxious, or depressed. This is commonly known as *social isolation*—physical separation and removal from the friends and family who know us, and on whom we can rely and trust, causing us great emotional distress. If any of this strikes a familiar note, this book is for you.

We weren't meant to live this way, in isolation. We were designed to be social beings, wired to seek out relationships with others and rely on them for communal protection and self-preservation, as Dr. Vivek Murthy reviews for us in his book *Together: The Healing Power of Human Connection in a Sometimes Lonely World* (2020). He reminds us that our earliest ancestors learned to recognize who around them is safe and trustworthy and who is a threat to be avoided. Ancient tribes and villages banded together and were there for one another in obtaining food, shelter, support, and protection, as well as in providing a community to help raise children and care for seniors. Forming relationships is a fundamental human need, an inborn matter of well-being and survival, and its essence continues to this day.

You can imagine that not having essential personal and social connections can feel devastating to a person. Social isolation puts us on guard, looking for constant threat; increases our vigilance; and affects our sense of safety, belonging, vulnerability, and anxiety. It's an unfamiliar and unpleasant experience that may result in physical and mental illness such as heart disease, stroke, obesity, sleep disorders, premature mortality, depression, anxiety, post-traumatic stress disorder (PTSD), cognitive decline, and other conditions.

Many factors can contribute to social isolation and loneliness. For example, in modern life we have drifted away from living in villages and small towns where the entire community looks out for and nurtures each other, and that has resulted in rising levels of seclusion and loneliness in our society. Many of us now live in big cities and may be far away from family, cautiously leaning on a few new, untested friends for support. In addition, our lives are affected by life transitions and disruptions; general medical events; race, ethnicity, and cultural issues; as well as preexisting mental health conditions—all of which can contribute to a feeling of isolation.

One example of events causing isolation in our current era has been the recent COVID-19 pandemic (caused by severe acute respiratory syndrome coronavirus 2, or SARS-CoV-2). COVID-19 has caused a worldwide health crisis that began in December 2019 and rapidly spread, with a major impact on us personally, medically, emotionally, socially, and economically. The threat of infection with this potentially lethal virus has caused us to change the way we live, significantly disrupting the lives and daily routines of all persons, whether or not infected. It's a cause of monumental stress, newfound fear, and anxiety in many. In response, most of us have dutifully remained at home, worked remotely when possible, homeschooled our children, wore face masks, followed handwashing guidelines, kept a physical distance from others, and limited the number of people who gather in any one place. In other words—we intentionally *isolated* ourselves.

There is a cost to living like this in a world of constant threat to our health and way of life, worrying about the health and well-being of our loved ones; managing the personal, financial, and economic challenges during these times; and watching it unfold in the media. Our relationships, sense of connectedness, employment opportunities, and social/recreational activities and interactions have suffered. Some of us have feared being in public places, work settings, shopping centers, and transportation systems, or medical center waiting, procedure, and exam rooms—all places where we might become infected during the pandemic. Others have, unfortunately, put off receiving medical evaluation, diagnostic tests, procedures, and treatment for their general health, resulting in a delay in diagnosis and treatment of potentially serious medical conditions.

While being alone for short periods can sometimes be restorative and helpful, unintentional or involuntary isolation often has a negative effect on our emotional health. Most of the life changes that accompany the COVID-19 pandemic have had a negative effect on our mental health and, similar to other infectious disease outbreaks requiring isolation, increased our levels of anxiety, loneliness, grief, depression, suicidality, PTSD, and substance abuse. We saw this in a survey of US adults done in 2018, before the pandemic, and again in April 2020, in which researchers found that levels of psychological distress and loneliness were higher during the pandemic than before (McGinty et al. 2020b).

Mental health symptoms may appear in those who have, or have not, been directly infected with or exposed to the coronavirus or encountered social isolation. Symptoms may appear in those who have, or have not, experienced a prior episode of mental illness. Some COVID-19 survivors may suffer short-term yet disabling mental health effects. In others, the impact can be long lasting, well beyond the physical effects of the virus or period of isolation, leading to PTSD and chronic mental health symptoms. Yet some experts predict that while the mental health effects of social isolation, and of the COVID-19 crisis in particular, will be significant, many persons will be resilient, able to cope with this stressor, and eventually recover naturally, moving on to a new normal and a satisfying life. *What's their secret?*

Understanding the mental health consequences of isolation and loneliness from all causes, including infectious disease outbreaks like COVID-19, enables us to help ourselves and others affected now in our current era and in the future. Many strategies can reduce both the short- and long-term distress caused by these events. That is the focus of this book, in which I present ways to recognize, prevent, and manage the mental health effects of social isolation along with interventions that have been of value during past events and are likely to be useful now.

How can this book help you? The aim of this book is to help you better understand the negative effects of isolation in you and your family, offer practical everyday mental health recommendations and self-care strategies for dealing with this, provide guidance on the major types of professional mental health care and mental health providers, and advise you on what to do when someone refuses treatment or has suicidal thoughts. It's a practical guide written for the general public with a focus on dealing with social isolation, using our collective experience of the COVID-19 pandemic and its effects on us as an example. This book is based on scientific literature and my interviews with clinical experts in the field: four actively practicing therapists, whose professional experiences and recommendations for dealing with social isolation are scattered throughout this book. In writing, I relied on these interviews and the scientific evidence to provide information useful to you in your daily life; it is not meant to be a comprehensive textbook on the subject.

One question I consider is, Why are some people more susceptible to emotional distress and develop a debilitating emotional response during or following social isolation while others seem to cope better and are able to move on? One answer, proposed by Southwick and Charney in their book *Resilience: The Science of Maintaining Life's Greatest Challenges* (2012), lies in building and maintaining resilience, which is the ability to bounce back after adversity and is covered in chapter 12 of this book.

In their work, Southwick and Charney learned that those who have resilience all tend to use the same or similar coping strategies during moments of high stress. The authors identified ten coping strategies that have proved effective in dealing with stress and trauma. These include confronting your fears; maintaining an optimistic but realistic outlook; accepting social support; attending to your own health and well-being, including physical exercise; and other factors. While this list may seem overwhelming, try not to worry if you feel you don't have strong resiliency skills right now. I will walk you through them and show you how, with a little effort and direction, you can improve your resilience.

Reconnecting after Isolation is divided into two parts. Part I covers how social isolation affects us. It begins in chapter 1 with a definition and an overview of isolation and loneliness and their impact on you, followed by the effect of social isolation on mental health, using the COVID-19 pandemic as an example. Chapter 2 covers emotional distress, functional impairment, and stress, and includes effective coping strategies for social isolation and for the pandemic in particular. In chapter 3, I present the concept of fear and effective steps to face our fears. Then fatigue and burnout are the focus of chapter 4, with helpful recommendations to avoid burnout. Next comes a discussion of bereavement and grief, with grief coping strategies for yourself and your children. Chapter 6 looks at how social isolation can affect our mental health and includes depression, anxiety, PTSD, and other conditions, along with a section on how to manage your mental health and deal with stigma. Chapter 7 explores suicidal thoughts and impulses, and chapter 8 is devoted to substance use disorder.

The focus of part II is on what you can do to help yourself. It begins with understanding the underlying basics of mental health in chapter 9. The basics are a series of daily steps we all need to maintain our emotional health and stability, including sleep, diet, exercise, having a routine and structure, and connecting with others. I encourage you all to increase your social supports and build structure and purpose into your day. This may seem like an overwhelming task to you at the moment, but it is possible to do if you approach it in small steps, one at a time.

Next, in chapter 10, you will learn about finding the optimal kinds of professional mental health providers and methods of treatment for you or a loved one, how to access them, how to tell if you're getting better, and what to do if someone refuses treatment or you cannot afford to pay for it. Chapter 11 explores various talk therapy options, or psychotherapy. Then in chapter 12 we look at building and maintaining resilience, which helps to control and stabilize our mental health. Finally, chapter 13 addresses reentry anxiety, the uneasiness we may experience upon returning to our usual daily life and activities after isolation, such as during the COVID-19 pandemic. The book closes with some final thoughts I have on mental health care and access.

I encourage you not to fear reaching out for professional mental health evaluation and treatment if you develop any prolonged emotional symptoms that last longer than two weeks, cause you distress, or interfere with your daily functioning.

Four mental health experts graciously agreed to be interviewed by me for this book and offered much valuable insight on the experience of social isolation and its treatment options. I am most grateful to them for their generosity and thoughtful contributions. My interview process was to speak with each person privately over Zoom, record our conversation with their permission, and take careful notes. Relevant sections from our conversation were then inserted into this book. These mental health professionals are

Thea Gallagher, PsyD
Director of Outpatient Clinic, Center for the Treatment
and Study of Anxiety
Perelman School of Medicine
University of Pennsylvania
Philadelphia, PA

Douglas Katz, PhD
Department of Psychiatry
Director of Psychology, Dauten Family Center for Bipolar
Treatment Innovation
Massachusetts General Hospital
Instructor in Psychology
Harvard Medical School
Boston, MA

Sheila Rauch, PhD
Professor, Department of Psychiatry and Behavioral Sciences
Clinical Director, Emory Healthcare Veterans Program
Emory University School of Medicine
Atlanta, GA
Board of Directors, Anxiety and Depression Association
of America (ADAA)

Wendy Silverman, PhD
Professor, Yale Child Study Center and Professor
of Psychology
Director, Yale Child Study Center Program Anxiety
and Mood Disorders Program
Yale University School of Medicine
New Haven, CT

PART ONE

How Does Social Isolation Affect Me?

CHAPTER 1

What Is Social Isolation?

I begin this book with the premise that we are all social beings and need personal connection with others to survive and thrive. Meaningful, genuine relationships are essential to our well-being and allow us to share purpose, interests, pursuits, and personal values with others. Getting together and interacting with our friends, colleagues, and family provides us with many benefits, such as a feeling of acceptance, increased self-esteem, a chance for friendship and fun, and access to someone who can provide support if we need it. This kind of social contact and support helps us maintain our emotional health and protects us from developing or worsening episodes of depression, anxiety, post-traumatic stress disorder (PTSD), and other mental illness. The opposite, social isolation and physical separation, is not healthy for us or our brains, and we flounder.

Social isolation can be brought on by changes in our personal life circumstances. Some experiences that can lead to social isolation include:

- *General medical events*: for example, social isolation occurs when we're stuck at home on crutches for months with a broken leg; confined to bed rest for months during a difficult pregnancy; after we've had a stroke or physical disability; when we're in the midst of certain cancer therapies; following a bone marrow transplant; or having physical challenges that limit our mobility, hearing, or vision.

- *Life transitions and disruptions*: we may feel more isolated when we lose a loved one, move to a new town or remote location, or retire from work; graduate into the elderly years or move to a nursing home; adapt to a pandemic such as COVID-19 and live with social distancing restrictions; become a victim of intimate partner violence; experience unemployment with associated perceived shame; and other life events.
- *Race, ethnicity, cultural, religious, and gender differences* can cause feelings of isolation and being left out of the mainstream of society.
- *Mental illness*: isolation is often associated with pre-existing depression, anxiety, social anxiety disorder, and other conditions. These can contribute to or be a result of social isolation and loneliness.

In a world where we depend on social interactions, we will nevertheless still spend some time alone, and all alone time is not the same. When our alone time comes from social isolation, it can have negative consequences on our physical and mental health and ideally must be avoided. Spending *some* time alone each day, however, without feeling lonely can be beneficial. *Solitude*, rather than isolation, has a purpose and is often soothing and rejuvenating. Solitude allows us to think, self-reflect, relax, and replenish ourselves, especially when we're overwhelmed. It's something we choose to experience, in contrast to the involuntary isolation of mental illness, a pandemic, or a major life disruption. We all need a bit of solitude or restorative alone time in our lives. A quiet walk outdoors alone in nature, meditation, prayer, art, music, reading, or working on a favorite hobby can be soothing and provide us with a sense of contentment, peace, and renewal.

Even though solitude is alone time, it is not the same as the isolation and withdrawal that comes with stressful life events.

Sometimes we are stressed and involuntarily find ourselves having to deal with social isolation, physically separated from others, including the friends and family we rely on and trust. It steals our sense of belonging and connectedness with those who know us well.

Social isolation is linked closely to *loneliness*. Think of loneliness as an overwhelming feeling of being cut off and apart from others, where no one knows you well, and you're unable to connect with them on a deeper level. Loneliness is sometimes referred to as *perceived social isolation*—our view or experience of being alone. It can occur regardless of who or how many people are included in your social circle or home life and can even be felt while you're in a crowd, on the subway, or in the classroom. And the reverse is true—a person can be physically isolated from others by choice, living a solitary life, and not feel lonely. For example, if you're a fisherman at sea for prolonged periods or a long-distance truck driver hauling goods, since it's your chosen life, you're likely to be content and not feel lonely.

Dr. Jeremy Nobel, of Harvard Medical School and the director of the UnLonely Project, defines loneliness as the "self-perceived gap between the social connections one wants to have and what one is actually experiencing" (Nobel 2021). Loneliness can affect us on many levels, causing both physical and emotional symptoms. It's often associated with psychological distress, increasing our risk of impaired mental health, depression, anxiety, suicidal behavior, sleep problems, disturbed appetite, and other symptoms. Feeling lonely can lead to a decline in our sense of well-being and our concentration, decision-making, and problem-solving abilities. Loneliness also has an impact on our physical health that is comparable to tobacco smoking, poor eating habits, obesity, and a sedentary lifestyle.

Perceived social isolation, or loneliness, may cause us to feel unsafe and hypervigilant, constantly on the lookout for new threats. We might view the social world as a menacing and frightening place and expect to have negative social interactions, further distancing ourselves from others and reinforcing our loneliness. Yet experiencing loneliness may also motivate us to connect more with others—this is one way we have adapted over the centuries to ensure our safety and survival.

There are thought to be three dimensions of loneliness, described by Dr. Vitek Murthy in *Together* (2020) and reported in the scientific literature. Experiencing any one of these can make us feel lonely:

- *Intimate or emotional loneliness*: longing for a close confidante or intimate partner
- *Relational or social loneliness*: yearning for quality friendships and social companionship and support
- *Collective loneliness*: desiring a network or community of people who share our sense of purpose and interests

Many things can contribute to our feeling isolated or lonely. It's believed to be a combination of our genes, past experiences, current circumstances, culture and community, and individual personality characteristics. Traditions and our culture affect the quality of our connections by shaping our social expectations and attitudes. Loneliness can occur when our lived experience fails to meet our social expectations for love, friendship, and community that are set by family, friends, schools, workplaces, neighborhoods, television, and media. For example, if a person has come to expect that they will have a spouse and children, they will likely feel lonely and distressed if that doesn't happen.

Loneliness had been increasing in our society even before the COVID-19 pandemic. For example, in a 2019 national survey of Americans, 61 percent reported feeling lonely, up from 54 percent in 2018 (Cigna 2020). The Cigna survey report noted the following factors contribute to loneliness:

- a lack of social support
- too few meaningful social interactions

- negative feelings about one's personal relationships
- poor physical and mental health
- a lack of balance in one's daily activities—doing too much or too little of any given thing (e.g., sleep, work)

Jeremy Nobel points out that stigma and silence make loneliness more difficult to deal with, and that some people are ashamed and embarrassed about being lonely. He writes that "many perceive loneliness as their own fault, attributable to falling short in some way, to not being worthy of friendship, attention, or authentic connection to others. Essentially, it's something to be ashamed of. As a result, many don't talk about their loneliness."

Those who live in cultures that promote self-reliance as a virtue have found this to be particularly true. For example, many adult men have been raised to appear strong and independent, as are many athletes, professionals, and certain societies and cultural or social groups. So, when they feel lonely, they struggle in silence.

THE RISKS AND IMPACT OF SOCIAL ISOLATION

An abundance of scientific literature describes the risks and impact of social isolation on our physical and mental health. Researchers have found associations between isolation and increased heart and cardiovascular disease, systolic blood pressure, cholesterol, mortality, inflammatory disease, weakened immune function, and impaired sleep. They have also found isolation-related increases in dementia and cognitive decline, stress and increased cortisol (stress hormone) levels, depression, anxiety, PTSD, suicidal thoughts, and other mental illness. Those experiencing loneliness are found to be less likely to be physically active or care for themselves and are more likely to smoke tobacco, be obese, and abuse alcohol, all leading to an increase in physical and mental health problems.

Social isolation and loneliness can have a negative effect on many areas of modern life. Two are explored below.

Disruptions in Daily Living and Routines

Social isolation strikingly changes our daily life and activities. Home, work, and social life suffer. Our usual patterns of sleep, diet, and exercise turn into late nights or interrupted sleep; grazing for food all day instead of eating three healthy meals; and exercise limited to walking around the neighborhood, if that. We may fear and avoid going to a restaurant, retail shop, church or synagogue, gym or exercise class with others so we remain at home.

During periods of social isolation, we often lack routine, structure, and purpose in the endless days of confinement—this presents a risk to our mental health. It's thought that disruption of our daily routine, even small changes, places stress on the body's ability to maintain emotional stability, and that those who have mental illness may have a more difficult time adapting to these changes in routine. Paying close attention to daily routines, and to the positive and negative events that influence those routines and cause us stress, increases our stability.

Social isolation affects the lives of many children and adolescents. They may be experiencing prolonged time away from their friends, teachers, relatives, extended families, and communities and are now living with uncertainty and unpredictability because of the pandemic, which most find difficult and disruptive. Children need to have structure and order in their day.

Social distancing and school closures have been found to increase depression, anxiety, and other mental health problems in this age group. Your child may be sad, irritable, hostile, and difficult to get along with, as well as having changes in their sleep, eating patterns, academic work, and circle of friends. Loneliness, particularly in childhood or adolescence, may be associated with future mental health problems, such as depression and anxiety, up to nine years after the experience. In addition, the length of time spent in isolation often predicts mental health problems in the future.

Having a purpose and direction in life is central to our wellness and well-being.

Many children living under isolation are homeschooled virtually, with parental supervision, *if* they have the required technical literacy, computer and software technology, and WiFi access. Remote education can present a challenge for children who have difficulty sustaining attention, especially when they are without social cues or reinforcement from the teacher or others. It also presents time management issues that are new tasks for them to learn. This can lead to frustration, anxiety, worry, and irritability. Of added concern is a recent NAMI Massachusetts panel discussion of college students and young adults that revealed many students tend to "zone out" and not pay attention during virtual classes on Zoom.

Some students attend school in a hybrid program; a few attend in person. Concerns are that their overall education might suffer, yet experts point out that most children are resilient and will eventually catch up. Socialization, physical activities, and sports are limited to backyard or street games with siblings, although a few risk participating in sports teams when available. Special needs students may lack the additional services needed to get through their day, which places an even greater stress on families who have to find a way to adapt.

In addition, many college students and twenty-somethings have returned to live at home during the COVID-19 pandemic, attending classes or working virtually from their childhood rooms or family basements. This has stretched some family relationships and caused additional layers of stress for both parents and their offspring, including younger children at home. While it may be tolerable in the short term, it affects the maturation and social development of these young adults, who would otherwise be out in the world learning how to make decisions and fend for themselves.

Being around your family full time, while you love them, can be stressful. Little things we do can become big annoyances or problems. When your children miss their friends and usual classroom, sports, and play activities, they quickly become bored and irritable, requiring you to be more patient and creative while managing your household and perhaps working from home. Sharing household and family responsibilities with your spouse or significant other, when available, is ideal, yet in reality, intimate relationships may be strained at these times.

Social isolation leads us to interact in new ways with our extended family, friends, and coworkers that may cause interpersonal tension, stress, and disagreement. "Modern progress has brought unprecedented advances that make it easier for us technically to connect," writes Vivek Murthy, "but often these advances create unforeseen challenges that make us feel more alone and disconnected" (Murthy 2020). During times of isolation, the in-person social experiences we had with friends and distant family are now mainly done virtually, except for those immediate family members who are in our "bubble" of safety. Many of us have become fatigued using technology for all our work and social interactions.

Even if a relationship was strong to begin with, the COVID-related stressors (health risks, finances, childcare, isolation, working remotely), combined with preexisting personal vulnerabilities (health, age, stage in life, mental illness, or trauma history), can affect how well couples communicate, problem solve, preserve their relationship, maintain previous activities, and manage the pandemic.

Dr. Wendy Silverman says that, for those children who have anxiety, going back to school after being home for one year (when socially isolated because of the COVID-19 pandemic) is a difficult situation. Being at home was initially a traumatic, unusual experience for them. Yet children and adolescents became very comfortable being at home; some have bonded more with parents and siblings, and suddenly, they're supposed to go back. It's hard for them to return to in-person school, particularly those whose bodies and psychological selves have naturally changed and matured over the past year.

Dr. Silverman explains that there's a relationship between early pubertal development and internalizing and externalizing problems such as depression, anxiety, and behavior problems (in other words, keeping your feelings inside versus expressing them openly). This makes the child more self-conscious and sometimes more irritable and hostile. She notes that this may occur more often in minority populations. There's also a realistic fear of teasing, bullying, and being made fun of because of an adolescent's physical changes. Some children are reluctant to return to school, and she has recently observed school refusal behaviors in her clinic. Dr. Silverman also notes that some parents, for example, Asian American parents, are reluctant to send their children back to school for fear of COVID-19 scapegoating behaviors and bullying that their children are likely to face.

Author interview with Dr. Wendy Silverman, March 8, 2021

For example, during the COVID-19 pandemic, couples and families have struggled over how strictly they should adhere to the social distancing guidelines from the Centers for Disease Control and Prevention (CDC), whether to contact or avoid other people or go to a restaurant, store, or sporting event. Dr. Karestan Koenen, a psychologist at Massachusetts General Hospital and psychiatric epidemiologist at the Harvard T.H. Chan School of Public Health, Boston, Massachusetts, has noted that "people are feeling isolated even with the people they live with, because there's a lot of stress and conflict" (as quoted in Sweet 2021).

Last, there are reports of an increase in domestic violence and child abuse during periods of isolation, including during the COVID-19 pandemic. Intimate partner violence (IPV) refers to physical, emotional, sexual, and psychological violence directed at a partner, such as a spouse. As people are confined to their homes with the stay-at-home orders, some IPV victims become trapped inside with their abusers. The pandemic-related economic impact of job losses, unemployment, closure or limited access to alternate housing (shelters, designated hotels), and travel restrictions have limited access to safe havens. Closure of schools and childcare facilities have compounded the problem, adding to an increase in partner and child abuse. During this time the number of calls to domestic violence hotlines has decreased, however, because victims have been unable to safely connect with needed services, fearing their abuser is listening in on their conversation, reading text messages or emails, and so on. Much needs to be done.

Disruptions in Work Routines

During periods of enforced social isolation, some of us are the essential workers who remain in their work setting; some may work from home; others have become furloughed or may have lost their job and are now in search of anything to pay the bills. Loss of employment and the way one sees oneself, being unable to support one's family as the breadwinner, often leads to a loss of self-esteem and self-respect and increased family tension.

For many of us who have jobs, physical isolation restrictions and guidelines require that we work virtually—on Zoom, Microsoft Teams, or the equivalent. We're challenged during this time in having to learn new work skills and adapt to new technologies such as teleconferencing. When working from home, the work-home-life boundaries often evaporate, and we find ourselves working more hours and taking fewer daily breaks. For example, ten months into the COVID-19 pandemic, workdays were still 10 to 20 percent longer than before. There are more late-night emails, meetings, and work procedure changes, and people are not

There is great financial uncertainty and struggle in trying to find work during these times of high unemployment, adding tremendous stress.

taking vacation or sick days. Spending the entire working day at home with our spouses, children, or aging parents means more distractions and disruptions, and many feel they are less productive. Some like working remotely, however, because of the flexibility it offers, with no time wasted commuting to work.

Working remotely can be isolating and lonely. Specifically, working remotely and relying on virtual communication has reduced our much-needed personal contact—less casual office chatter flavors our day. We lose that spontaneous in-person interaction that can lead to important outcomes at work, sharing knowledge and creating new ideas, innovations, and collaborations of benefit to organizations in the future. This means that managers and employees have to work harder during the pandemic to build and maintain informal bonding and relationships among workers, which help improve communication among them. It now all has to be done at the "virtual watercooler."

And then, when working from home remotely, we now have to deal with *Zoom fatigue*, the new phrase for the tiredness, worry, or burnout associated with overusing technology for virtual communication. This experience has become common during times of social isolation, including during the COVID-19 pandemic. It's exhausting to participate in multiple video meetings and teleconferences each day. Many of the normal nonverbal visual cues we rely on during in-person conversation are not obvious virtually, such as making eye contact and observing hand gestures, body language, posture, and subtle signs that someone intends to speak. It takes more effort to concentrate on the message because there's a millisecond audio delay in the conversation between speakers, which alters our perception. We also have to remember to "unmute" before we speak. I'm guilty of that!

> Dr. Thea Gallagher observes that because of social isolation in most of our work relationships, we're not making small talk. We're not getting a lot of positive validation, feedback, and acknowledgment that we get just being in the office, seeing people, sharing a joke, or connecting in other ways. She reflects that "even though many of us work from home and we might spend all day talking to people, I think we can feel isolated because we aren't connecting in our humanness in the same way that we used to. And so work feels very much like we're kind of robots."
>
> Author interview with Dr. Thea Gallagher, January 15, 2021

Parents working from home have competing interests between home and work responsibilities and supervising their children's lives and interrupted education, including virtual classroom activities and homework, playtime, sports, and exercise activities, all while ensuring their healthy socialization and development. Many find this overwhelming, leading to feeling guilty and that they've somehow failed in these areas of life. Parents—married and single—find themselves juggling the demands of their working lives with their parental, family, and household responsibilities as the new normal, feeling as though there is no end in sight. This all contributes to fatigue, anxiety, and depression.

EFFECTS OF QUARANTINE

In our discussion of social isolation, it's of value to include the concept of *quarantine*, which is the physical separation and restriction of movement following an infectious disease exposure while waiting to see if the person becomes ill. It is done to reduce the chance of someone infecting other (healthy) people and carries many negative mental health effects. Being in quarantine adds to our stress because of being strictly separated from loved ones, confined to home with the loss of usual routines and the freedom and ability to go places, having reduced social and physical contact, uncertainty over personal health status, fear of infecting others, anger, frustration, and boredom.

The length of time we're quarantined has a negative impact on our mental health, resulting in exhaustion, anxiety, irritability, poor sleep, difficulty concentrating and making decisions, post-traumatic stress, and anger. A longer time in quarantine is related to more intense emotional symptoms, adding to psychological distress.

MENTAL HEALTH CONSEQUENCES OF SOCIAL ISOLATION

Dr. Sheila Rauch emphasizes *isolation* as the biggest issue affecting mental health today; many other experts agree with her. During and following social isolation, those who have no prior history of mental health problems may experience psychological symptoms for the first time. Those who experience a first episode may not recognize their symptoms, often lack the skills necessary to manage their illness, and may be currently without treatment, struggling on their own. In those instances, a person may not know what is bothering them, the importance of seeking treatment, what kinds of treatments are available, and how to access needed mental health care services.

Social isolation also affects those of us who already have a preexisting mental health condition and who may or may not currently be in treatment. The effects of isolation and social distancing may potentially worsen our prior psychological symptoms. The impact is more profound in those of us who already experience anxiety, depression, bipolar disorder, or other mental illness.

Researchers have looked at the impact of social isolation on our mental health. They learned that being flexible in our thinking, tolerating uncertainty, and accepting difficult experiences appeared to act as a buffer against the negative effects of increased social isolation.

SOME EXAMPLES OF SOCIAL ISOLATION AND LONELINESS

Certain infectious disease outbreaks that have occurred in the world have led to the experience of social isolation. These outbreaks, called either an *epidemic* or a *pandemic*, are ongoing events lasting many months (or longer) with long-term effects on individuals and society. They are:

- Ebola virus,
- SARS (severe acute respiratory syndrome),
- MERS (Middle East respiratory syndrome),
- H1N1 (swine flu), and
- COVID-19 (from severe acute respiratory syndrome coronavirus 2, or SARS-CoV-2).

There is a commonality in the effect these events and their associated isolation have on our lives and in our reactions to them, leading to similar personal, social, economic, and emotional pain and suffering. Reports of increased anxiety, depression, and PTSD have followed these infectious disease outbreaks.

The Example of COVID-19

Let's now look at the experience of the COVID-19 pandemic as an example of social isolation and loneliness. In December 2019 the first cases of a new (novel) coronavirus, severe acute respiratory syndrome coronavirus 2 (SARS-CoV-2), which causes COVID-19, were reported in Wuhan, China, and rapidly spread to create a worldwide pandemic lasting through 2020 and into 2022. The short- and long-term physical, emotional, societal, and economic burden of this illness has been immense, shutting down major cities, countries, and economies in its wake.

Infection with the novel coronavirus is spread person to person through respiratory particles or droplets when we speak, cough, sneeze, or sing. The greatest risk is exposure within less than six feet. It has also been spread through eye secretions when we touch our face and eyes. It's easy to understand the risk and fear of contracting the virus from someone who has physical symptoms of the illness—we become aware of them and know not to get close.

A pandemic is the worldwide spread of a new disease, essentially an infectious disease outbreak that spreads to more than one continent; most people do not have immunity.

Yet, it's been estimated that more than half (59 percent) of those who are infected with the COVID-19 coronavirus are without symptoms (asymptomatic) and may spread the disease to others without knowing; other researchers believe that it's hard to estimate these numbers.

The most common initial symptoms of coronavirus infection are fever, chills, cough, sore throat, fatigue, muscle aches, and sometimes nausea or diarrhea. Some experience a loss of smell or taste. Severe symptoms include shortness of breath, rapid progression of respiratory failure and acute respiratory distress syndrome (ARDS), requiring a mechanical breathing tube in an intensive care unit (ICU). Groups at increased risk of experiencing severe illness are the elderly, those residing in nursing homes and close quarters (prisons, rehabilitation facilities, group homes), and those who have a preexisting medical condition such as diabetes, heart or lung disease, cancer, or obesity.

Most people are able to recover at home. For those who are ill or in the hospital receiving supportive care, the Food and Drug Administration (FDA) has given emergency use authorization for an antiviral medication (Remdesivir, in November 2020), monoclonal antibody treatment (in October 2020), and convalescent plasma (in August 2020). While these therapies have been effective, infection with COVID-19 still carries an increased risk of early death. For example, almost one-third of 1,648 patients who were admitted to several hospitals in Michigan for COVID-19 died during hospitalization or within 60 days of discharge (Chopra et al. 2021). The most effective approach is preventive, with a vaccine targeted to the COVID-19 virus; at this writing, several effective vaccines are now available throughout the world, and the process of administering them to everyone 5 years of age or older has progressed. It's not yet clear whether this will be a one-time or annual vaccine shot, as genetic variants to the COVID-19 virus have been identified, and a fourth surge of infection has begun in Europe and the United States.

COVID-Related Life Changes
In general, COVID-19 has had a major impact on us medically, socially, and economically, with significant disruption to our lives and daily routines and a loss of normalcy. This disruption includes our relationships with loved ones, friends, and communities; daily home, work, and social routines; cultural and religious customs; work and recreational activities; and our livelihoods. Dr. Koenen describes the pandemic as unpredictable, a threat to us and our loved ones that initially (until we get the vaccine) we feel a lack of control over. Some people have been unfairly

blamed by others for creating the virus (notably those of Asian descent) or for contracting and spreading it, leading to stigma.

During the pandemic we are obliged to follow safety and preventive guidelines regarding our behavior in an effort to contain spread of the virus. Following social distancing guidelines and COVID-19 restrictions is a matter of personal responsibility. The response of most governments and communities to the COVID-19 pandemic has been to treat those affected with supportive care and treatment as described above and to minimize spread of the virus while scientists work on developing and distributing an effective vaccine. Their recommendations for containment of the virus include wearing a face mask to protect ourselves and others, fastidious handwashing, keeping a distance of six feet or more between individuals (social distancing), and limiting the numbers of people gathering in one place at a time to a minimum. Yet this has led to a *loss of normalcy*, with changes affecting all aspects of our lives—how we work, go to school, interact with other people, shop for food, mail something from the post office, engage in recreational activities—everything. While designed to keep us safe, the restrictions placed on us to contain the COVID-19 virus have had a severe impact on our mental health.

At times during the pandemic, communities, schools, businesses—retail, restaurant, hospitality, and service—recreational activities, health clubs, and religious institutions have had to completely shut down. Graduations, proms, weddings, funerals, and other milestone and significant occasions have had to be cancelled or modified because of the pandemic. Our usual grief and bereavement customs and rituals have also been greatly altered, leading to feelings of guilt and difficulty reaching closure.

In the first surge of infection, lockdowns and stay-at-home orders were in effect in many states and countries. Many people were furloughed, laid off, or told to work remotely from home.

It left numbers of us out of work, affecting our personal financial savings and ability to cover daily expenses; education was interrupted; and the economy fell rapidly in a downward spiral. There have been varying degrees of opening back up in stages or phases, only to shut down again during the second and third surges of the pandemic in the fall of 2020 and winter 2021—and again later in 2021 and in 2022 in places.

Many of us found ourselves juggling work, home duties, family, and children from home. Having competing interests and responsibilities has become the *new normal* for many working and single parents during the pandemic. For example, some parents have struggled with work and household duties while supervising their young children's virtual classroom activities and homework, playtime, sports, and exercise activities, all while ensuring their healthy growth and development of social skills. Many find this overwhelming, leading to feeling guilty and that we've somehow failed in these areas of life. Please see chapters 2 and 4 for more on maternal depression and parenting.

Many people understand the challenging situation pretty well; others feel anger, frustration, and resentment because of interruptions to their lives and goals. During the COVID-19 pandemic, many of us have confined ourselves to home, supermarket, and pharmacy. Yet a sufficient number don't follow the guidelines, resulting in a repeat surge of infections worldwide, especially following the 2020 holiday season.

Some experts believe that we will see a partial, not complete, eradication of COVID-19 as a result of persons failing to follow the recommended preventive guidelines, including refusing to receive the vaccine, or due to genetic mutations of the current virus causing variants. We may also experience other pandemics in the future. All of this will continue to affect our physical and emotional selves, requiring us to pay close attention to those at increased risk for mental health conditions with more aggressive mental health screening, evaluation, treatment, and public education.

Work Changes

As a result of the nature of their jobs, and out of fear of losing highly valued employment and income, some have been forced to go to their usual workplace during the pandemic—these are the essential workers in hospitals, grocery stores, pharmacies, public service agencies, and transportation systems. If you're an essential worker—thank you! Essential workers continue to do their jobs at times like these, physically showing up at work to sustain us. Yet they come home in fear of having been exposed to the virus and potentially infecting their families.

Others have experienced major changes in their work life as they work remotely from home, are furloughed, or have lost their job and are now searching for a way to sustain themselves. A Pew Research Center survey found that one-fourth of US adults reported layoffs or job loss in their household because of the coronavirus outbreak, and about one-third reported pay cuts in their household due to reduced hours or demand for their work. Forty-two percent have experienced one or both of these. Job losses and pay cuts were especially common among younger adults, Hispanics, and those in lower-income families. Difficulty paying bills and financial and food insecurity were more common among adults with lower incomes, those without a college degree, and Black and Hispanic Americans (Parker, Minkin, and Bennett 2020).

Working remotely from home has required a great deal of adjustment from workers and has affected their productivity and relationships with colleagues and family members. Some good has come of learning that remote working is entirely possible; it can decrease the organization's costs of providing work spaces and employees' commuting time and expenses, as well as increasing their availability for family members. The future likely holds a hybrid model in the workplace with a combination of in-person and remote working.

Access to Health Care

During the COVID-19 pandemic, many changes have occurred in our health care systems. The massive numbers of people affected by the pandemic has strained, sometimes surpassed, the capacity of health care services and hospitals in most countries. A survey conducted by the World Health Organization (WHO) among the health officials in five WHO regions in May–July 2020 found disruptions of essential health services in nearly all countries (more in lower-income countries). Seventy-six percent reported a decrease in outpatient visits and elective procedures (WHO 2020).

Other changes included staff reassignment or redeployment from other clinical departments to care for COVID-19 patients, unavailability of some services due to facility or health clinic closures, and difficulties obtaining equipment for staff (personal protective equipment, or PPE) and for patients (respirators, ICU beds, etc.) through the supply chain. In response, many have made adjustments using triage of health services, telemedicine outpatient visits, and changes in dispensing approaches for medicines.

Many people have put off preventive medicine visits and getting essential screening exams and evaluations for fear of contracting the virus at the medical center or clinic. Unfortunately, this reluctance to seek medical care raises concerns of delay in diagnosis and treatment for other medical conditions such as heart disease, stroke, and cancer.

A lot of us have taken to telemedicine (virtual clinical appointments on a computer) during the pandemic. We like having to take less time off from work to see a clinician with essentially no commute times. It's worked pretty well for most types of medical appointments. Reliance on telemedicine, however, creates a problem in access to health care, as some people do not have the technology (computers and WiFi) or technical skills (technical literacy) to engage in a virtual appointment. The overall goal post-COVID is to resume in-person appointments and necessary procedures, with telemedicine use as an alternative. Please see chapter 10 for more on telemedicine and telehealth.

Many of us have felt great fear of becoming infected when entering hospitals and medical centers or clinics during the pandemic.

Dr. Sheila Rauch has been working on telehealth research for many years, particularly as it applies to the treatment of PTSD. She sees it as a way to improve access to mental health care, getting treatment out of the clinics and directly to the patients. In her work she has found that telemedicine treatment is equivalent to face-to-face treatment for a few mental health interventions, and she has good evidence of most patients experiencing the same outcomes with both approaches. Dr. Rauch has observed that for most people who have PTSD, depression, or other mental health disorders, telehealth is a good option and, in many ways, can be better. Nonetheless, she has seen patients vary a lot in how comfortable they are in using this technology.

Author interview with Dr. Sheila Rauch, December 21, 2020

Economic Changes

COVID-19 has led to changes in the economy, with a major impact on our personal finances, which are being spent down, and on the world economy, which has lost a significant portion of retail, restaurant, and travel and hospitality business. Prior socializing with friends and family in restaurants and cafes is now being done virtually, except for those immediate family members who are in our "bubble" of safety. Recreational activities, health clubs, religious institutions closed—then opened partially—and closed again. Manufacturing and retail has slowed down because of a global supply chain crisis, with delays in acquiring raw materials and serious transportation issues; at this writing there are hundreds of container ships in the harbor waiting to be unloaded and transported.

So far, the total cost of the COVID-19 pandemic is estimated to be $16 trillion in the United States alone, with about half of this due to lost income from the COVID-19-induced recession and the remainder from the economic effects of premature deaths (due to a shorter and less healthy life). The pandemic is associated with job loss, furlough, or mandatory working from home with potentially less productivity; spending down of retirement and savings funds; loss of health insurance, particularly following a job loss; risk to maintaining homes with subsequent fear of eviction; insufficient funds to pay for food, with food insecurity leading to widespread dependance on food banks; increased reliance on virtual systems for work, classroom education, and telemedicine globally, limited for some by lack of technical literacy and access, as well as other factors.

Mental Health Consequences of COVID-19

Most of the life changes that accompany the COVID-19 crisis have a negative effect on our mental health, our ability to manage it, and the stabilizing factors in our lives that support our emotional health. They include:

- social isolation with limited in-person human contact and support, including mental health clinicians and peer support groups;
- increased fear and anxiety about becoming ill (self or family);

- lack of routine, structure, and purpose in the endless days of confinement;
- variations in routine sleep, dietary, and exercise habits;
- new sources of major stress and uncertainty;
- societal and personal financial losses; and
- increased anxiety, which already occurs in 50 percent of those who have depression.

COVID-19 presents many valid reasons for us to feel distressed, fearful, and lonely, beginning with the need for social isolation and quarantining. We're lonely because we're forced to take specific actions (isolation and restrictions) to protect ourselves in response to a common enemy—a potentially deadly virus.

In previous coronavirus respiratory outbreaks (such as the 2003 SARS epidemic) depression, anxiety, and PTSD were each observed in about one-third of survivors at six months and beyond following infection. Most experts believe that similar instances of prolonged or chronic mental health symptoms will also occur following COVID-19.

It's been found that those exposed to or recovering from infection with COVID-19 have an increased risk of depression, anxiety, PTSD, and substance use. This is true whether or not we have been directly infected with or exposed to the virus. For example, increased risk of mental illness may follow direct contact or exposure to the infection if you've contracted the virus, or from indirect contact through the pandemic's effect on our loved ones and communities and living in a high-risk COVID-19 area surrounded by the virus. This is not unusual following such exposure.

One survey of random US adults reported that the percentage of depression symptoms was three times higher in 2020, during the COVID-19 pandemic, than in 2018, before the pandemic (Ettman et al. 2020). In addition, the CDC's Household

Pulse Survey (CDC 2021) suggests that the percentage of US adults with symptoms of anxiety disorder and/or depressive disorder has quadrupled since before the pandemic.

Dr. Sheila Rauch describes the COVID-19 pandemic as an insidious exposure similar to that of military soldiers in combat (deployment) for 12 to 18 months. In both situations, there are

- *chronic, continuous, underlying stress: as during combat, the novel coronavirus has created an increased sense of threat to all our lives daily, with a focus on our keeping safe and changing our behavior (e.g., wearing face masks, social distancing, self-isolation at home);*
- *periodic and specific "punches" of trauma along the way (personal illness, death of a loved one, loss of job or home, financial losses, etc.);*
- *social isolation; and*
- *loss of resources and removal of previous supports.*

All of this has an impact on the body and brain and increases our risk of mental health problems, including depression, PTSD, or substance use.

On top of that, other life situations happen; some people have lost economic resources, stability, their role in life when losing a job or income, and more. These are high-risk factors for having a negative mental health outcome.

Author interview with Dr. Sheila Rauch, December 21, 2020

It's helpful to identify who among those persons are at greater risk for infection and are more vulnerable to COVID-related mental illness. A review of the scientific literature published in 2021 found that depressive and anxiety disorders increased globally during 2020 due to the pandemic, with higher rates in females and younger age groups (COVID-19 Mental Disorders Collaborators 2021).

The CDC published the results of a 2020 survey of US adults that showed increased symptoms of anxiety, depression, substance use, and suicidal thoughts during the pandemic (Czeisler et al. 2020). More than 40 percent of adults experienced serious mental health problems, 13 percent increased drug or alcohol use because of pandemic stress, and 11 percent had serious suicide thoughts in the 30 days prior to the survey.

The number of calls to a suicide and help hotline in Los Angeles, California, increased from 22 calls per day in February 2020 to 1,800 calls per day one month later.

Those at increased risk included young people (who are often in life transition), racial and ethnic minorities, essential workers, and caregivers of adults. Risk and vulnerability can also come from having a preexisting medical condition, lower socioeconomic status, or being put in harm's way as an essential worker. For a summary of the findings of this survey, see table 1.1. These results are supported in a follow-up survey of US adults in the latter half of 2020 into 2021, when more young adults reported feeling anxious or depressed approximately five months after the COVID-19 lockdowns were imposed, and fewer reported getting the mental health counseling they needed.

As mentioned earlier, mental health symptoms may appear in those of us who have or have not experienced a prior episode of mental illness. Those of us who have a preexisting mental health condition may struggle more during the pandemic and find a worsening of our symptoms.

Yet some predict that while the mental health impact of social isolation, and the COVID-19 crisis in particular, will be significant, many persons will be resilient, able to cope with this stressor, and eventually recover naturally, moving on to a new normal and a satisfying life. It's been observed during the pandemic that some of us who have an existing mental illness appear to do fairly well, in part because we've already learned the necessary CBT and coping skills in therapy required to manage the illness during these times (Gallagher interview). These skills enable us to process our emotions surrounding the isolation and what we've been through and move forward with our lives. Since we may not always be able to access these mental health skills, however, many continue to struggle. Others may learn from their experience and grow as a result, something called post-traumatic growth (PTG), discussed in chapter 6. Those who are not able to process their emotions or grow from it may go on to develop PTSD.

TABLE 1.1 US Centers for Disease Control and Prevention 2020 Survey of Adults

- Mental health symptoms were higher in essential workers versus nonessential workers. (Essential workers are nurses, doctors, other health care workers, first responders, factory workers, hospital custodians, grocery store clerks, etc.) Many don't have job security and risk their health and the health of their families to meet basic needs.
- More than half of essential workers reported at least one adverse mental or behavioral health symptom, and 22% reported suicidal thoughts.
- Symptoms of anxiety, depression, and substance use were greater in Hispanics than whites.
- Thoughts of suicide were significantly higher among Hispanics (18.6%) and Blacks (15.1%) than among whites (7.9%).
- About two-thirds of unpaid caregivers for adults reported at least one adverse mental or behavioral health symptom.
- Three-quarters of those age 18–24 reported at least one adverse mental or behavioral health symptom. Serious suicidal ideation among this group was 25%.

Source: Czeisler, 2020.

> Dr. Douglas Katz and I spoke of the effects of COVID-19 on those who have a preexisting mental health condition. He has observed that some people become overwhelmed and anxious in having to comply with the CDC safety guidelines (face masks, etc.) and restrictions and with the uncertainty, panic, and fear of this crisis. Some have been unable to focus and work at their usual jobs because of this. That's been distressing to those who have worked so hard to rebuild their lives.
>
> Dr. Katz has seen people who had been doing well with their mental illness before the pandemic, with meaningful lives, unravel in their personal progress during the pandemic. Several have now slipped back into episodes of depression or mania and find themselves struggling and unable to continue using virtual technology to connect with him. Treatment has required a lot of work in therapy. Dr. Katz emphasizes thinking about these situations as "a setback that occurred in the context of extraordinary circumstances" and not as permanent evidence of being unable to function or care for themselves.

Author interview with Dr. Douglas Katz, December 28, 2020

CHAPTER 2

Stress and Coping Skills

The life disruptions and health-related risks caused by social isolation, including isolation caused by the novel coronavirus (COVID-19) pandemic, are challenging and can cause us daily stress. Social isolation can lead to depression, anxiety, loneliness, stress, burnout, grief and prolonged grief response, and PTSD. Most of the life changes that accompany social isolation and the pandemic have a negative effect on our mental health, our ability to manage it, and the stabilizing factors in our lives that support our emotional health.

Some persons may be more susceptible to stress during social isolation or an infectious disease outbreak, such as those who have prior mental health conditions. For example:

• Preexisting anxiety and worry is worsened by the uncertainty and threat of infection.

• Fear of contamination in those who have OCD (obsessive compulsive disorder) is amplified by the need to wear masks, wash hands, and keep a social distance.

• Loneliness and isolation in those who struggle with depression is increased by the loss of or decrease in social connections during these times.

Most people who feel bad want to know, "What's wrong with me?" or "Am I mentally ill?" I urge you to be cautious against labeling every emotion you feel as "abnormal" or as a "mental health problem," especially those emotional responses most of us would assume to be natural and expected following social isolation or a pandemic. Emotional distress is very real and expected at these times, and people are understandably troubled, but we may not *always* reach the level of clinical depression or anxiety and may not *always* need professional mental health treatment. Some of us will have sufficient resilience and coping skills to weather the crisis. When in doubt, discuss your symptoms of emotional distress with your primary care provider (PCP).

EMOTIONAL DISTRESS AND IMPAIRED FUNCTIONING

Any changes from your usual baseline self that interfere with your ability to function in daily activities (work, school, family, social) and that last two weeks or longer may be of concern and indicate significant emotional distress. Some of these include irritability, sadness, anxiety, excess worry, grief, guilt, anger, intentional withdrawal and isolation, hopelessness, suicidal thoughts, and multiple physical complaints (headache, muscle aches, nausea, heart pounding, gastrointestinal symptoms like nausea, vomiting, or diarrhea). You may experience fatigue; changes in energy level, sleep, or appetite; lack of interest in doing usual activities; or unintentional weight loss or gain. Some people might feel numb or disconnected. Others may experience reduced productivity, struggles in getting along with others (interpersonal conflict), trouble concentrating or thinking, memory lapses, and difficulty making decisions. The key is whether or not you have *functional impairment* in daily life—an inability to go about your usual daily activities and responsibilities.

In children and adolescents, it's recommended that parents pay particular attention to any problem their child shows in daily functioning at home, school, and in family or social relationships and consider it a sign of emotional disturbance and *potential* mental illness in their child. The most common sources

of impairment (that are not directly connected with a mental
health diagnosis) are parent-child relationship problems, sibling
and peer relationship problems, low-level disruptive behavior,
and work or academic performance issues. *Functional impairment* in a child or an adolescent can lead to an increased risk
of continuing emotional problems and mental health disorders
in the future. In a well-regarded 1999 study, researchers found

*In her specialty clinic, Dr. Wendy Silverman sees many
children, adolescents, and families who experience anxiety. She recommends that if a child is struggling with anxiety,
COVID-related fears, and other causes of emotional pain, a parent
be on the lookout for impairment in functioning and whether
their child is experiencing distress.*

*"We want our children to be able to developmentally progress
when it comes to their academic work, peer relationships, and
how they interact and deal with the family . . . and to deal with
their own personal distress." She describes an impaired child as
one who "is not going out because they're so afraid. That's affecting them in going to school, or they're not able to interact with
their peers, or it's prohibiting the family from engaging in family
activities. So [she encourages parents and providers to] consider,
how is [the child] feeling? Is he or she distressed?"*

*Dr. Silverman uses the acronym FISH to determine a child's
level of impairment and whether they need professional mental
health treatment. F stands for frequency of mental health symptoms; IS for intensity and severity of symptoms; and H for how
long it's been going on. When the Yale Child Study Center evalu-
ates impairment, they use a "feelings thermometer or an impairment thermometer [with ratings] from zero to eight."*

*Dr. Silverman also explains to children how they could have
or experience something but that it may or may not cause impairment.*

Author interview with Dr. Wendy Silverman, March 8, 2021

that many children and adolescents who experienced clinically significant psychological and social impairment were not found to meet the full criteria in the *Diagnostic and Statistical Manual of Mental Disorders* for any psychiatric diagnosis (Angold et al. 1999), leading to potential undertreatment of severe symptoms.

WHAT IS STRESS?

Stress is an emotionally and physically disturbing experience or condition you may have in response to changing and challenging life events, such as living and managing your life during periods of social isolation or a pandemic. And when you're also suffering from depression or anxiety, dealing with stress can become more difficult to handle. It can also make your depression, anxiety, or PTSD worse and contribute to relapse (a return of symptoms).

Stress can come from events inside or outside you. The causes and intensity of stress may vary from person to person, but common causes include:

- real events in life (positive or negative, marriage, divorce, birth, job, finances, a major loss, social isolation, or an infectious disease outbreak)
- relationships
- an illness, such as an infectious disease during an outbreak like COVID-19
- change of any kind, in home, lifestyle, work, social situations
- balancing work, family, homeschooling, and childcare during social isolation
- working remotely from home
- your environment
- overload of responsibilities at home and work
- an unresolved conflict

- a situation not under your control, such as imposed social isolation or a pandemic
- uncertainty while waiting on an unknown outcome, for example, a new COVID vaccine and possible eradication of the virus
- other stressors

Symptoms of Stress

We naturally have a *fight or flight* response inside our bodies (in our autonomic nervous system) that is turned on during times of stress. The fight or flight response leads us to be on guard and ready to fight, along with an assortment of unpleasant physical and emotional symptoms.

Physical symptoms of stress include general muscle and joint aches and pains, headache, chest pain, rapid heart rate, fatigue, trouble sleeping, upset stomach, and others. Stress can also cause symptoms of emotional distress, anxiety and panic attacks, depression and sadness, sometimes accompanied by excess drinking, gambling, eating, shopping, or sexual activity.

Sometimes our fight or flight stress response is turned on when we don't really need it, causing us unnecessary distress.

You can actively take steps to lessen the effects of stress and decrease your vulnerability to stressors. This is called *coping*. When you manage stress using effective coping strategies, you decrease the negative effect that stress has on your body.

EFFECTIVE COPING SKILLS

As you read this book, you might be wondering how to care for yourself in the stress and aftermath of social isolation or during the restrictions or quarantine period of a pandemic. Here are some suggestions that many people who face this have found to be effective. They include coping skills to manage stress, parenting tips, helping your adolescent and teen, practicing mindfulness, strategies to use in response to social isolation and COVID-19, and managing remote working from home and Zoom fatigue.

What Are Coping Skills?

Coping skills are the actions we take to lessen the effect of stressors and get us through difficult times. You can learn to do these skills on your own and apply or modify them for your children. They include problem solving, self-soothing, distraction, relaxation, humor, and managing the little things before they get too big. Learning and using effective coping skills are essential to managing living in social isolation and with the COVID-19 pandemic.

Coping strategies include ways to prevent and prepare for stress as well as skills for managing it when it occurs. Here are some approaches that many have found useful:

1. Maintain a regular schedule and structure of activities. This includes optimizing your sleep, diet and nutrition, exercise, and self-care.
2. Manage the little daily stressors.
   - Prioritize your responsibilities and activities.
   - Keep yourself organized.
   - Maintain a schedule but don't overschedule; adjust as needed.
   - Learn to say no on occasion.
   - Break down large or complex tasks into smaller pieces that are more manageable.
   - Keep a to-do list and a daily reminders list.
   - Write things down in a notebook, including health care–related questions and instructions.
   - Use a daily pillbox for your medications to keep track of when/whether you took them.

- Develop a system that you like and that works for you to manage the mail, bills, and housekeeping.
- Avoid overstimulation if possible.
- Be mindful, in this moment.

3. Use cognitive behavioral therapy (CBT) strategies. A life event can cause stress depending on how we interpret it, what spin we put on it. Usually, we interpret events based on our individual beliefs and past experiences. Sometimes we also interpret events with unintentional distortions in our thinking (negative, all-or-nothing black-and-white thinking, etc.). Challenging these distorted thoughts and interpretations using CBT can affect the way we feel and respond and can improve our level of stress.

- Keep a journal of your thoughts and feelings.
- Identify the sources of your stress. This will help you respond to it in a more effective way, when you know what you are dealing with.
- Be assertive in your communication—this helps you feel in control of your situation.
- Keep your perspective.

4. Use problem-solving strategies.

- Speak with someone (a friend, therapist) for help as you work out a problem.
- Get accurate information about the problem to make an informed decision.
- Evaluate and define the situation realistically.
- Consider your options and the alternatives.
- List the pros and cons of your options.
- Seek additional assistance as needed.

5. Distract and refocus your attention.

- Occupy your mind with other thoughts and activities—this temporarily takes you away from the stressor or problem at hand. Try puzzles, reading, hobbies, sports, gardening, or other things you like to do. Keep in mind, though, that this is not a permanent fix.

Wow—this is a lot! But you don't have to do all of these at once—try one or two at a time and see what works for you.

- Volunteer your time; reach out to others. You get back more in return.
- Replace your current emotion with another (e.g., by watching a movie or reading a book that's funny or scary).
- Leave the situation aside mentally for a while.

6. Try relaxation techniques (work with your therapist to learn these skills).
   - Progressive muscle relaxation—relax each muscle in your body from head to toe, one muscle group at a time (start with your jaw, then move to your neck, shoulders, arms, fingers, etc.).
   - Visualization—sit and focus on a calm, serene image or a place where you feel relaxed.
   - Biofeedback—discuss with your therapist how to learn this technique.
   - Meditation—Herbert Benson's book *The Relaxation Response* (2001) gives detailed information on getting started.
   - Deep breathing exercise—sit quietly and focus only on your breathing, taking slow deep breaths. Do this for 3 to 5 minutes. If your mind wanders, refocus on each breath.

7. Use humor: watch a funny movie on Netflix or DVD, read a funny book or the comics. Being able to appreciate humor is a healthy coping strategy.

8. Use self-soothing strategies—comfort and nurture your-
self with gentleness and kindness, using the five senses.
   - *Vision*: enjoy looking at flowers, art, or other objects
     of beauty; visit museums; get out in nature; see a
     play, musical, or dance production on TV now and
     in person when the pandemic clears.
   - *Taste*: enjoy a favorite food or beverage; take it slow
     and savor the experience.
   - *Smell*: use a favorite fragrance or lotion; buy flowers
     or walk through a flower garden or shop; bake cinna-
     mon rolls or cookies.
   - *Touch*: take a bubble bath, get a massage (but not
     during COVID), wear comfortable fabrics.
   - *Hearing*: listen to beautiful, soothing music or
     sounds of nature; sing; play an instrument.
9. Use mindfulness techniques (see below)

MINDFULNESS

Mindfulness is a way of living your life by focusing on the present moment. It's a way of *being* in the world, adopted from
Eastern meditation practices. The skills learned in mindfulness
practice have been found helpful in managing anxiety and mood
disorders.

As described by Jon Kabat-Zinn (1994), mindfulness means
being in the present moment in a particular way by
   - paying attention
   - on purpose
   - nonjudgmentally

Being in the present moment means that instead of being
preoccupied with the past or future, you are focused on and attentive to the present, what is happening right now. This is not
easy to do. It is common for the mind to wander, particularly to

thoughts of past events or future worries. The key is to notice when your thoughts drift and then bring your mind back to the present. Becoming so deeply involved in doing something that you lose track of time is an example of being in the present moment.

Mindfulness is a skill where you . . .

- Focus on the present moment, on purpose, nonjudgmentally.
- Do one thing at a time, in just this moment.
- Avoid ruminating about the past or worrying about the future.

Mindfulness requires that you pay attention to what is going on around you. It means that you live with awareness instead of going through life on autopilot. Paying attention also involves observing your own thoughts and feelings, your body's response to emotion (such as rapid heart rate, sweating, etc.), your urges, and your behaviors just as they are.

Being nonjudgmental means that you avoid being critical or making any judgment about your own thoughts, actions, or experiences. Let each moment be as it is. Allow yourself to think or feel what you are feeling, without putting labels or judgment on it. Often, part of your mind is constantly evaluating your experiences, comparing them to past experiences or expectations you may have. Instead, work on developing a neutral attitude toward what comes into your mind without judging it. Acknowledge your thoughts as thoughts and then let them go.

For each experience, emotion, or thought you have, try to feel it without reacting to it. Here's one way to try it. Imagine yourself sitting in a car on a foggy day, with the windshield wipers going slowly. Each stray thought is like a leaf that lands on the windshield. Allow the wiper blades to brush the leaf aside and in this way clear your mind.

Why Practice Mindfulness?

- Living mindfully allows you to engage in what you are doing. Emotions will interfere less often. This will improve the quality of your life.
- Mindfulness helps you to live in the present moment instead of experiencing painful emotions related to the past or future. Dwelling on past experiences or future worries tends to trigger painful emotions. This happens often in depression. Mindfulness practice helps you to decrease these ruminations and the emotions and distress they produce.
- Mindfulness practice can help you manage your mood disorder and anxiety. When you have increased awareness of the present moment, you are able to notice when these symptoms arise. Recognizing your symptoms enables you to respond effectively with a relapse prevention plan.
- Mindfulness can improve your ability to tolerate and respond to painful events. When you are overwhelmed by emotions, your mind clutters up quickly. So you have to focus first on the thought or moment and try to clear your mind, to calm it down. To do this you must step back, observe your own thought, and try to get a handle on it. Mindfulness practice can help you do this. When you are focused on and attentive to the present moment, without attaching judgment or value to it, you can make the best use of your thoughts, take action, and work on your problem.
- Many people find that mindfulness-based cognitive behavioral therapy is an effective treatment for anxiety and depression.

How Do You Practice Mindfulness?

Mindfulness is a skill that you can develop with practice. Begin by trying to make yourself more aware of the present moment without judging it as good or bad. Focus your full attention on what you are doing, on one thing at a time. Get fully involved in that moment. Notice when your mind wanders and bring your attention back to the moment. You can begin to practice this by setting aside 5 minutes a day to do a mindfulness meditation (see below).

You can also try to exercise mindfulness as you go about your day. For example, when you brush your teeth, focus your mind on doing only that one task. Pay attention to your actions, to the taste, sensations, sounds, and so on. As your mind wanders, bring it back to the task of brushing your teeth in this moment. Try it again when you drive, wash the dishes, have a conversation, or during other moments of your life. Live with awareness of what you are doing instead of going through life automatically.

Exercise to Practice Being Mindful

1. Sit in a comfortable chair, in a comfortable position.
2. Close your eyes if you like.
3. Become aware of your breathing and focus on each breath.
4. Anchor your attention to the present moment: pay attention to your breathing, the sounds around you, the physical sensations you have.
5. Observe what you feel, see, and hear without placing a value or judgment on it.
6. Continue to focus on each breath, in and out.
7. When intrusive thoughts come into your mind, let them go without judging them or yourself. Return your focus to your breathing. Over time it will become easier to focus your mind in this way.

VALUE OF PETS IN HELPING YOU THROUGH ISOLATION

Many households in the United States have at least one pet, which can provide us with a lot of health benefits. Pets give us unconditional love, warmth, loyalty, companionship, connection, social support, and a sense of purpose, particularly in seniors. They can help us be more social, for example, as we come to meet new people when out walking and playing with our dog. Caring for a pet also gives us a reason to get out of the house and in the fresh air.

Owning a cat or dog can help raise our energy levels; reduce mental fatigue, stress, anxiety, loneliness, and depression; lower our risk of social isolation; and encourage exercise and playfulness. Pets provide us with calming support and a routine, and caring for them can be a distraction from upsetting symptoms or experiences; they also have a role in behavioral activation (see chapter 11). One research study found that pet owners experienced a greater sense of well-being and had healthier personality characteristics, and that pets complemented other forms of social support (friends and family) rather than competing with them (McConnell, Brown, and Shoda 2011). Evidence for the role of pets in those who have a mental health condition, including therapy pets, is still early, although it is thought that effects would be similar to those in the general population.

The CDC reports studies showing that the bond between people and their pets can increase fitness, lower stress, and bring happiness to their owners. Some of the health benefits of having a pet include:
- decreased blood pressure
- decreased cholesterol levels
- decreased triglyceride levels
- decreased feelings of loneliness
- increased opportunities for exercise and outdoor activities
- increased opportunities for socialization

COPING STRATEGIES DURING SOCIAL ISOLATION AND COVID-19

The social isolation we may experience as a result of the COVID-19 pandemic carries with it a unique set of stressors and occurrences. We need to respond to these in effective ways in order to cope and manage them. This section presents some thoughts on coping strategies that have been found useful during isolation. I begin with suggestions offered by Dr. Thea Gallagher.

In our interview Dr. Thea Gallagher spoke of the many people who feel like they're failing at everything during the pandemic—home life, parenting, managing homeschooling and children's recreational activities while working, work life, new job, relationships, self-care, and other areas. In fact, they have been given impossible choices with competing interests to navigate with no ideal solution. She suggests that we create healthy boundaries, daily structure, and routine, and maintain good self-care. Ask for help when needed and work out a division of labor with your partner for household and childcare responsibilities. Give yourself credit for what you are doing and take some time for yourself.

Author interview with Dr. Thea Gallagher, December 16, 2020

As Dr. Gallagher points out, parenting issues and skills is one of the many areas of concern during these times. In a recent *Harvard Business Review* article (Dowling 2020), the author addressed the issues of working parents who are fraught with feelings of guilt and failure as parents, as well as their own personal loneliness. Dowling recommends setting work-home boundaries and being direct with your supervisors at work regarding the competing obligations you have at work and at home with childcare or elder care. Some have found that a working parents' network or support group is helpful.

There is strong support for two strategies found to be effective in preventing or minimizing mental health symptoms like depression or anxiety during these times: *maintaining social connections* and *physical activity.* Below you will find some other ways to handle the stress and any symptoms you or your child may have. They will enable you to cope more effectively and bounce back more readily from the medical, social, emotional, and economic threats of social isolation and the COVID-19 experience.

Accept and adapt. Those who accept the reality of their situation—social isolation or the COVID-19 pandemic—and adapt to their new life circumstances (social distancing, working from home, etc.), while continuing with the things in life that provide meaning and purpose, have a greater chance of maintaining emotional stability.

Stay intentionally busy. Stay busy in a meaningful way. Predictable and regular daily routines help keep our body's internal clock running smoothly, which is important to our well-being. Having structure, meaning, and purpose is key. Prioritize all the things that you need to get done. If you feel overwhelmed and disorganized, try writing everything down in a list and then create a schedule.

Try to keep up with your regular family, household, personal care, and work routines and responsibilities. Focus on what's important to you. Think about different pursuits you can work on, for example, connecting with others; cleaning and organizing your home, closets, or drawers; working on your hobbies and projects; or learning something new from a free online class. If you have children, remember that they're used to routine and structure in school, homework, sports, and social activities. Consistency helps them feel in control and less anxious, which in turn can calm you.

Connect. Make an effort to reach out to others with creative use of social media, by phone or videoconferencing (FaceTime,

Skype, Zoom, etc.), or in person with those in your bubble of safety. Be imaginative and plan special activities, like playing a musical instrument or a board game with friends over social media, or having regular "Drinks in the Driveway" get-togethers with friends and neighbors—just remember to maintain social distancing and don't overdo the alcohol.

Use your proven coping strategies. Humor, hobbies, pets, music, and exercise all help in managing depression and anxiety. Aim for a relaxation routine or yoga (online or on your own) and pleasurable moments in each day. Try to do things with family at home or with friends virtually, such as games, exercise, music, funny movies, yardwork, or cooking and baking. There is more on this later on in this chapter.

Focus on the moment, what you can do now. Give yourself credit for what you are able to do now, even if it's little things. Put aside the regrets and what-ifs. Try not to make comparisons to the way your life was or what you would prefer it to be—these situations are most often temporary, and you'll have plenty of time to get back to your previous, or newly prioritized, lifestyle and pursuits.

Care for yourself. Attend to your personal care each day: shower, shave, wash your hair, and get dressed in clean clothes instead of staying in your PJs or sweats all day. Make your bed. Make *real meals* for yourself with real food. Take your prescribed medications as directed—getting a 90-day supply will decrease your anxiety about running out. Make an effort to avoid or limit alcohol, street drugs, tobacco, and excess caffeine.

Get regular sleep. Go to bed and get up at the same time each day, maintaining a steady sleep pattern. Staying up late or having fragmented, erratic sleep will only worsen your symptoms. Avoid daytime naps—they tend to interfere with nighttime sleep.

Feed your body; feed your brain. Your brain needs fuel to operate. Eat three healthy meals at the same time each day instead of snacking or grazing all day on junk food or skipping meals. This will stabilize your blood sugar, which then has a positive impact on mood and brain functioning. Ideally, enjoy your meals with another person, even if it's virtually or on social media.

Move more, sit less. Exercise is an excellent way to maintain mental and physical health. It increases a chemical called BDNF (brain-derived neurotrophic factor) that acts like brain fertilizer to grow new brain cells and multiply the connections between them. During this time, try to stay as physically active as possible and spend some time outdoors each day getting fresh air. Walk the dog; play tag with your kids; go on a fitness walk or run; steadily climb up and down two flights of stairs in your house or apartment building for 20 minutes straight three times a week (the low-tech StairMaster); do stationary floor exercises like leg squats, leg lifts, jumping jacks, and sit-ups. Gretchen Reynolds, a *New York Times* journalist, has written many articles on fitness and physical health; I highly recommend one called "The Scientific 7 Minute Workout" (Reynolds, n.d.).

Home environment and activities. Keep your home environment fairly organized, tidy, and clean. Clutter can cause you to feel uneasy and lethargic, and the worse it gets, the harder it is to find things and eventually clean it up. Do the laundry, fold it, and even bring out the iron, which I'm told is a soothing ritual for some. Be creative in planning family and social activities.

While it's not easy to do, set home/work boundaries and take periodic breaks from work for your mental health. Work as a team with everyone in your household and expect your children to participate and do their part in maintaining the home environment in an age-appropriate way. Set clear guidelines, basic rules, and a schedule for everyone to follow. Be sure to include time to care for those who depend on you (children, seniors) as well as time for your own self-care and work responsibilities. Pace yourself.

Stay informed. Learn about what's currently happening in your world—natural disasters or the coronavirus pandemic and its complications—without becoming obsessed or overwhelmed by it. *Limit* your news exposure to one brief period once or twice a day to keep current in this rapidly changing environment. Avoid accessing the news at bedtime because that will be overly stimulating and may interfere with your sleep. Get accurate facts from reliable sources and be wary of different versions posted online or on social media. Be aware of misinformation circulating about. For example,

- Search out experts who use well-accepted scientific methods to analyze the data and publish their results in reputable medical journals.
- Pay attention to those organizations whose mission is to inform and protect the public, such as the CDC and the WHO.
- Avoid sources who try to promote or sell a product related to the information they provide.

Manage your mental illness. Watch for the onset of or worsening symptoms of depression or anxiety. Mindfulness techniques that focus on the present and CBT strategies designed to address negative and distorted thoughts, inaccurate beliefs, and unhelpful behaviors often improve depression and anxiety symptoms. Reach out to others through online support groups and chat rooms. The Depression and Bipolar Support Alliance (DBSA) and the National Alliance on Mental Illness (NAMI), national mental health support, advocacy, and educational organizations with local chapters, have recently been facilitating groups online and through Zoom.

If you have an established mental health diagnosis, stay in regular touch with your mental health treatment team, ideally through virtual appointments (telemedicine) on a computer or by telephone. Make sure you always have an adequate supply of your prescribed medications and try to adapt the skills you learned in therapy to this new life circumstance. If depression is a new experience for you or you don't have a mental health clinician, contact your family doctor for evaluation and treatment recommendations.

If you're in crisis or having a mental health emergency, contact your health care provider directly to evaluate your current symptoms and determine the best course of action. If you don't have a PCP or a mental health clinician, call your hospital's Department of Psychiatry or Emergency Department to see if they have established an outpatient urgent care mental health clinic where you can be seen and evaluated. If you are suicidal, call your provider or 9-1-1 immediately for assessment and treatment or go to the Emergency Department.

> **COVID Coach app**: COVID Coach is a free, easy-to-use, evidence-based mobile app from the VA National Center for PTSD, with self-care strategies designed to promote health and wellness for anyone affected by the COVID-19 pandemic (available through Apple's App Store, https://apps.apple.com/us/app /covid-coach/id1504705038, or through Google Play for Android devices). The app includes brief, simple tools and resources for coping, mindfulness, stress, sleep, mood and anxiety management, and wellness. The National Center for PTSD also provides other self-help, education, and support apps for PTSD, mindfulness, CBT for insomnia (CBT-I), and other areas (VA Mobile Apps, https://www.ptsd.va.gov/appvid/mobile/index.asp).

HELPING YOUR CHILD COPE

During periods of stress brought on by social isolation or the pandemic, children's lives are disrupted and affected greatly. Your children may be without the usual structure and routine that is essential to healthy development and a sense of security. They may also be without their friends, teachers, relatives, extended families, and communities that support them. Create a daily routine for your children and pay attention to the positive and negative events that influence these routines and may cause stress. Set the expectation that they will follow it. Routines should include sleep, healthy diet and nutrition, physical exercise, helping out around the home with age-appropriate chores, and essential time connecting with others, even if it's on social media for now. While schoolwork is a priority, make sure that your children have enough social connection, creative outlets, play time, and physical activity. Pay attention to and limit the time your child or teen spends online, in computer games and on social media sites, and replace it with other activities. This may take the form of family games, kickball or soccer in the backyard or at an outdoor park, riding a bike, art or music projects, learning a new skill, caring for a pet, reading together, and other healthy pastimes that attract your children's interest and attention. Make sure your children know you're available to talk; answer their questions and address their fears and anxiety about what's going on around them.

MANAGE REMOTE WORKING FROM HOME

Working from home remotely has become common during periods of social isolation and the COVID-19 pandemic, but it can also be a source of great stress. An article in the *Harvard Business Review* (Rothbard 2020) offers some suggestions to deal with working from home in a virtual world.

- Create distinct boundaries with your time, with clearly designated work and home, family, and relationship time. Turn off work in your head during your at-home time. For example, you might decide to check work email messages only during official work hours; stop working

at a specific time each night; dress up for working remotely in Friday-casual work clothes—this will help you
separate work from home.

- Stick to a schedule of set working hours that can be modified if family matters arise. Inform your coworkers and
family members of your available time—your work time.
Take periodic breaks from work for your own mental
health.

*Dr. Thea Gallagher emphasizes the importance of separat-
ing work and home life, having strong work-life boundaries, and taking vacation days. She notes that during the pandemic,
"People weren't taking their vacation days because there's no-
where to go! [Everyone's saying,] 'Let me save them up.'" She goes
on to say that if you don't try to get to the core of what's going
on and take breaks, time off (including vacation days), and separate from work when you're home, you might end up even leaving
a situation, such as quitting a job, that actually could have been
modified.*

*"We need to take our vacation days, separate from our elec-
tronic devices, disconnect from our phones when we're not working, change our technology practices—it's really important to do
that." She also points out, "Leadership needs to adjust the expectations and stop pushing people to do more or even to just do the
same that they were doing before, because we're all managing a
much higher workload just because of the nature of this all . . .
I think also, though, we have to call on the management to [pro-
vide] technology resources and other kinds of support for people
who work from home."*

*Dr. Gallagher believes that we can't just be saying, "Yeah, it's
hard. Go take a yoga class." We really need to be talking about
these issues, educating people about what they're feeling and
experiencing.*

Author interview with Dr. Thea Gallagher, December 16, 2020

- Try to be fully present and aware when at work and also when you're with family and loved ones. It helps to try to clear your head at the end of the workday so you can accomplish this.
- Have a designated work space at home. It could be a corner of a room or a separate room if you have the space. Avoid bringing work papers or projects into the middle of your household if possible, which can blur the boundaries and make work seem never ending.
- Focus on improving communication with coworkers. Work to build and maintain relationships. This takes greater effort when working remotely since the opportunities for casual chatter are not available. Be creative in setting up a "virtual watercooler," which just means planning specific times virtually to get to know each other and share ideas.
- Clear up any questionable issues with your supervisor regarding work goals and tasks.

How to Handle Zoom Fatigue

Zoom fatigue is a type of mental exhaustion, worry, or burnout that you may feel from the increased demands and overuse of virtual communication techniques, such as video conferencing on Zoom or Microsoft Teams. It's related to our having to focus more attentively on the speaker and conversation to absorb and process information and having to stare continuously at a computer screen without any visual or mental break. Here are some suggestions on how to deal with Zoom fatigue.

- Stick to your daily routine—work time, evenings, and weekends should all be and feel different.
- Disconnect from technology regularly and when you need to.
- Try not to schedule back-to-back virtual meetings— plan for another activity in between calls.

- Avoid multitasking.
- Build in breaks during the day.
- Take a break from video—switch to phone calls or email.
- Practice mindfulness.

CHAPTER 3

Facing Our Fears

The COVID-19 pandemic experience is a cause of enormous daily stress, fear, and anxiety in many. Fear is an emotional and physical response triggered by the perception of some direct threat to ourselves. It's considered an adaptive response to danger in that it helps us gather our inner resources and deal with the potential threat. In response to this fear we might experience constant worry, trouble concentrating, intense emotions, impulsive reactions, sleep problems, racing heart, trembling, dry mouth, or sweaty palms.

When the threat is uncertain and ongoing, as in the COVID-19 pandemic, fear can become chronic and interfere with our daily functioning and quality of life. This can then affect our mental health and overall sense of well-being. In a 2020 survey (Fitzpatrick, Drawve, and Harris 2020), those who reported more fear and worry, seeing COVID-19 as a threat to themselves or their family's health, were more likely than others to report depressive and anxiety symptoms.

Fear leads to a set of behaviors beyond our typical ones. Some of these are safety measures that can lessen the fear or threat, such as wearing a face mask or frequent handwashing. But sometimes fear leads to an excess of these activities, such as watching news reports nonstop on TV or the internet; avoiding all social contact in any form; refusing to get a new physical symptom looked at by your physician; panic buying in a frenzy and hoarding goods (toilet paper and Clorox disinfectant wipes, for example), which then negatively affects the supply chain, making these items even more scarce.

How close we live to a coronavirus hotspot may influence how we experience and report specific feelings of fear, stress, and anxiety, and what preventive steps we may take in response. For example, researchers found (Fitzpatrick, Drawve, and Harris 2020) that the Northeast United States was consistently highest in reporting feelings of a perceived threat (fear) during the pandemic. This was thought to be related to the higher number of COVID-19 infections in that geographic area than in other parts of the country and world at the time. They also found noticeable differences in perceived threat between the Northeast and the Midwest United States, which had seen a smaller number of COVID-19 cases reported at the time of their survey.

Some examples of COVID-19 related fears and concerns include:

- *Fear of the unknown.* The COVID-19 coronavirus is a new virus never before seen in humans. The rate of infection, the course of the illness, potential treatments, and short- and long-term effects and outcomes are not known. We are just now observing and learning about the long-term consequences of the illness, such as residual heart, lung, joint, and mental health conditions.
- *Fear of not knowing who among us are* asymptomatic *persons*, those who have the virus but have no symptoms and from whom we could potentially become infected.
- *Fear of the staggering mortality rates.* The rate of COVID-related infections and deaths appears to be very high.
- *Fear of ourselves or loved ones contracting the virus, with uncertain and potentially fatal outcomes.* Most people fear becoming ill themselves, of not being able to breathe, or of being admitted to a hospital or ICU, reliant on a breathing tube without our loved ones nearby. We fear

dying prematurely and alone. The news reports flood us with visions of patients in hospital hallways with insufficient medical supplies and staff, along with daily statistical reports of premature deaths in all age groups.

- *Impaired ability to help loved ones or to grieve their loss.* We fear and regret being unable to help our family and loved ones if they do become ill; initial regulations prohibit us from seeing them in the hospital, allowing only virtual visits on a tablet computer if we're lucky. We fear living the experience of others whose loved ones passed away without them being present or able to say goodbye, attended to in their final moments by compassionate strangers. We mourn the loss of friends and family without being able to see them or to plan and attend a funeral or memorial service.
- *Fear of receiving the vaccine.* Since the COVID-19 virus is new to humans, the vaccines created to prevent its infection are also new (CDC 2021). Two main types of COVID-19 vaccine have been developed. One that uses new technology, called an mRNA vaccine, differs from others in that it does not contain the virus (and thus cannot "give" a person COVID). These are the vac-

Vaccines work by stimulating your immune system to create antibodies to a virus such as the coronavirus that causes COVID-19.

cines made by Pfizer-BioNTech, Moderna, and others. A second, more traditional type, called a viral vector vaccine, uses genetic material from the virus piggybacked on to a modified version of a second virus (the vector); it cannot infect you with either virus. These are made by Janssen/Johnson & Johnson, AstraZeneca, the University of Oxford, and others. Other COVID-19 vaccines are in development. As new vaccines, however, some people may regard them with a degree of uncertainty about their safety and effectiveness, especially since they were developed, produced, and approved in record time. Some persons may not trust the government and wonder if shortcuts were taken, even though we are reassured by the FDA that this did not happen. We don't yet know just how long the vaccines will be effective or if we'll need annual booster shots. Some wonder about the long-term side effects of the vaccine, and its effects on those who were not in the first clinical trials, such as young children and pregnant women.

• *Anxiety about changes in daily life.* The pandemic has disrupted work, school, family, social and recreational activities, with interruptions in education for children and some adults, as well as parents having to oversee home-schooling, all with a lack of structure and purpose.

• *Uncertainty about our lives.* What will happen to us, the impact this pandemic will have on our lives, is not clear to most of us. For the past 24-plus months, we have experienced major changes in our daily routines, how we relate to others and go out in the world, our jobs, schools, businesses, and recreational activities. We might be working from home remotely or working in a high-risk environment; our financial savings are diminishing; we might be supervising the virtual education and activities of our children from home; we are advised, sometimes mandated, to limit our social contacts, wear face masks, wash our hands, and keep a physical distance from others; we feel isolated; trips to the supermarket feel risky. We don't know how long these changes will be required and what life will be like as we try to resume normal activities. This uncertainty is a source of great anxiety.

- *Increased stress from restrictions.* We face restrictions on how we interact with others and the world, including how many people can gather in retail, restaurant, transportation, and religious venues, increasing our stress.
- *Loneliness due to social isolation and physical separation.* Human interaction has become much more challenging during the coronavirus pandemic, with limited in-person human contact, including with family, friends, coworkers, mental health clinicians, and peer support groups. The situation requires that we be creative and determined in finding opportunities for socialization. If not, the result of prolonged isolation is often greater depression, anxiety, or PTSD.
- *Concerns about insufficient access to both routine and urgent health care, treatments, procedures, medications, and resources.* Routine health care services have changed during the pandemic (Patel et al. 2020; WHO 2020). Some services are not offered during this time— for example, elective procedures. Many dentists' and eye doctors' offices were closed for several months at the beginning and are now open with different routines for safety. Some outpatient appointments are available virtually—a new experience for patient and provider. So far, in developed countries, routine medications have been in sufficient supply, and many persons elect to have them delivered to their homes rather than risk entering a pharmacy.
- *Fear and anxiety related to erratic changes in our econ-omy.* Job losses, changes, or furloughs and diminishing personal financial resources and sense of security are all sources of anxiety. For some people, this situation has led to an inability to pay basic bills, fear of eviction from homes, food insecurity, loss of job-related health

insurance while unable to afford private-pay health care services, and other financial losses.

All of this makes most of us uncomfortable. We don't know what to expect or how we will end up. The nearly continuous media coverage magnifies our fears, especially when varied, uncertain, rapidly changing, or contradictory information is circulated.

FACING FEARS

It's important to face any fears you might have so that they do not interrupt your functioning, the quality of your life, and your ability to experience pleasure. Here are some steps you can take to deal with the COVID-19 pandemic and its stressors, putting you in control so that your life is not driven by the fear:

- *Educate yourself about the virus.* Stay informed with reliable sources of information. Focus on the *facts.* Obtain evidence and professional opinion from trustworthy sources: the CDC, WHO, or a press report with Dr. Anthony Fauci, director of the National Institute of Allergy and Infectious Diseases (NIAID). You may want to share accurate information with family, neighbors, friends, and coworkers.
- *Monitor and limit your news exposure.* Even though news stations broadcast almost 24/7, it is not healthy to be continuously exposed to negative information. Limit your time spent watching the news on TV or reading news on the internet and in print to brief moments (5–10 minutes) once or twice a day.
- *Understand your risk for infection and put it into perspective.* This includes the impact of any underlying medical conditions you may have—asthma, heart disease, diabetes, immunosuppression from chemotherapy drugs, and so forth. If in doubt, discuss your risk with your

Steps to Facing Your Fears
1. Have a goal and focus on it.
2. Get reliable information about what you fear.
3. Think about how the fear makes you think and feel (this will help you understand its effect on you so that you can then take steps to manage it).
4. Consider the costs and benefits to you of addressing your fear instead of remaining in your comfort zone.
5. Develop a plan with small steps to deal with the fear.
6. Identify what kind of support you need and who will provide it (family, friends, colleagues).
7. Take the steps you have planned.
8. Assess your progress and modify your steps as needed.

Adapted in part from S. M. Southwick and D. S. Charney, *Resilience: The Science of Mastering Life's Greatest Challenges* (Cambridge: Cambridge University Press, 2012), section on Special Forces SERE School, pp. 56–62.

physician to get a realistic sense. Then, while taking the necessary protective precautions, put that worry aside and try not to obsess about it.

- *Know your underlying mental health conditions and the tools to manage them.* Learn about your anxiety, depression, or other mental health conditions and use the psychological tools you learn in therapy (like CBT skills and mindfulness) to help you cope with and contain your emotional response to the pandemic.
- *Keep connected with friends and family members.*
- *Have a daily routine and structure to your day.* Include pleasurable moments.
- *Separate your work and home life.* If you work from home, or are searching for a new job, designate a specific time and a separate place or corner in your home for

work-related activities. Hold yourself to the time frame
of reasonable work hours. Set boundaries for yourself
and your supervisor.

- *Do the same for your children's schooling.* Keep their virtual
classroom activities scheduled at discrete, specific times
and places in your home with necessary boundaries.
- *Take periodic breaks in your day.* This applies to adults
and children.
- *Get outside, preferably in nature.* Walk around the block,
play with your kids or dog, get a change in scenery.

CHAPTER 4

Fatigue and Burnout

FATIGUE AND MENTAL HEALTH

Fatigue is a symptom commonly found during periods of social isolation from any cause, including COVID-19 restrictions. It's also considered a core symptom in mood disorders, anxiety, and PTSD, affecting more than 75 percent of people who have major depression. Fatigue can significantly impair our ability to function and carry out our daily tasks. It may make it more difficult to get out of bed, get dressed, care for yourself or your family, prepare meals, perform household and family tasks, or get to work (even virtually). We may feel fatigue even when we think we are getting enough sleep, which can be quite frustrating.

What exactly is fatigue? There is no single definition. It is different from just feeling sleepy or tired. Fatigue can be thought of as a combination of symptoms, with three main parts or dimensions: physical, mental, and emotional. You may have several of these together. The multiple components of fatigue have been described in this way:

Physical
- loss of energy
- heavy limbs
- persistent tiredness even without physical exertion
- exhaustion
- reduced activity tolerance
- decreased physical endurance, stamina

- increased effort required to accomplish physical tasks
- generalized weakness
- slowness or sluggishness

Mental and Cognitive
- mental dulling
- word-finding and recall problems
- problems focusing and sustaining attention
- difficulty concentrating
- decreased mental endurance
- slowed thinking

Emotional and Psychological
- lack of motivation
- apathy, decreased interest
- weariness
- irritability
- boredom
- low mood

The fifth edition of the *Diagnostic and Statistical Manual of Mental Disorders* (*DSM-5*) describes the various dimensions of fatigue in its definition of depression, including physical fatigue (loss of energy), mental fatigue (difficulty concentrating), and emotional fatigue (loss of interest and pleasure, called *anhedonia*).

Fatigue has various possible causes, such as social isolation, stress, depression, or anxiety, which may be difficult to sort out. But it is important to identify which one applies to you, if possible, so that you and your health care provider can address and treat the problem of fatigue effectively. For example, fatigue can be a result of social isolation and of living through a pandemic or under excess stress. Most people feel overwhelmed, balancing many areas of life under unusual circumstances just to keep going. It can be complicated by boredom and being unable to participate in prior social, recreational, work, and family activities because of social isolation and quarantine.

Fatigue can be a primary symptom of depression, along with feelings of low mood, sadness, or loss of interest. Often this type of fatigue improves along with treatment for depression. But fatigue can also be a leftover or residual symptom of depression, persisting after treatment in about 23 to 38 percent of people who are otherwise in remission. (Nierenberg 1999, 2010). This means that, in some people, fatigue lasts even after most other depression symptoms have improved or gone away following treatment with antidepressant medication. Residual fatigue can be difficult to resolve, but therapeutic options are available—speak with your psychiatrist if you are having persistent fatigue.

Next, fatigue can be a side effect of medications, particularly some antidepressants, like SSRIs (selective serotonin reuptake inhibitors). Sometimes this requires a change in medication to a different drug with fewer side effects, one that you tolerate better. Discuss medication changes with your treating physician. Remember to be specific about your side effect symptoms and how they affect the quality of your life.

Fatigue can also be related to insomnia and poor sleep patterns, which often occur along with the stress of social isolation, COVID-19, depression, anxiety, PTSD, and other mental health conditions. If this is a cause of your fatigue, CBT-I (cognitive behavioral therapy for insomnia) and adhering to good sleep hygiene practices will benefit you.

Finally, fatigue may be related to other medical problems you may have. These problems may include diabetes; low thyroid condition; kidney, liver, lung, or heart disease; or others. These conditions do not necessarily cause the fatigue; there is just a potential association. In these cases, work with your treating physician to optimize your other medical conditions as much as possible.

What Helps with Fatigue?

Begin by considering the conditions that may be contributing to your fatigue and work with your PCP or mental health provider to modify what you can. In some cases you may need to avoid those medications that are apt to worsen sleepiness and

Get some exercise even when you're dragging and fatigued and don't feel like it—you'll be surprised how much it will improve your energy level.

fatigue, choose alternative medications more likely to help resolve the symptoms, or consider using an additional medication that targets fatigue. Discuss these options with your psychiatrist.

Next, stick to the basics of mental health covered in chapter 9 of this book. Remember to have nutritious meals on a regular basis, follow a consistent sleeping and waking pattern (with a goal of getting 7–8 hours of sleep per night), take your medications as prescribed, avoid alcohol and illegal substances, maintain a daily routine and schedule, and keep up with social contacts. Then, even though it sounds difficult, get out and exercise a little every day, at a moderate level, based on your current ability.

BURNOUT

Another experience you may encounter is burnout, which is not uncommon for those stretched thin living in social isolation, such as through the COVID-19 pandemic. Many people are trying to be and do everything for everybody at home, school, work, and in relationships, and this can lead to burnout. But what exactly is burnout?

Burnout refers to a kind of fatigue, the sense of having reached the limits of your endurance and your ability to cope with a situation. Burnout is the result of too many demands on your strength, emotional reserves, time, and energy, with a lack of resources and support. The situation goes beyond your ability to deal with it. Burnout has been associated with many physical and mental health conditions such as heart disease, high blood pressure, sleep problems, depression, anxiety, and alcohol or substance abuse.

The term *burnout* has most often been used to describe work-related experiences. It has three dimensions: exhaustion (see components of fatigue above); a feeling of being detached or distanced mentally from work or what you're doing, with cynicism and not caring; and a sense of incompetence, ineffectiveness, and lack of accomplishment (efficacy). In 2019 burnout was officially recognized by the WHO in its International Classification of Diseases (ICD-11) as an occupational phenomenon, but not a medical condition, in the chapter "Factors Influencing Health Status or Contact with Health Services." They defined it as "a syndrome . . . resulting from chronic workplace stress that has not been successfully managed" and specified that the term should not be used to describe events in other areas of life (WHO 2019).

Some experts differ in its use and strive to redefine burnout as "the mental and physical impact of accumulated stress in any sphere of life" (McBride 2021), and "the impact of chronic exposure to emotionally draining environments" (Rionda, Cortés-Garcia, and de la Villa Moral Jiménez 2021). Burnout has been a common experience among caregivers, such as parents (called *parental burnout*) and health care workers, and in those enduring the stressors of managing a chronic illness or experiencing social isolation and the COVID-19 pandemic, where every aspect of life has required additional effort. Parental burnout may leave people feeling trapped, unable to leave their responsibilities and take time off or a vacation. Some parents may even become co-ercive, punitive, neglectful of, or violent toward their children (Abramson 2021; Griffith 2020; Mikolajczak et al. 2018). This is where mini-breaks or moments to pause are invaluable.

When experiencing burnout, you may feel a combination of physical and emotional symptoms, such as:
- frustration, irritability, or anger
- sadness, depression
- disinterest, apathy, indifference—lacking feelings, finding it more difficult to empathize with others
- resentment or pessimism
- isolation or disconnection from others
- the need to self-soothe with alcohol or street drugs
- recrimination—blaming of self or others
- helplessness—feeling like a failure, that nothing you do can help
- headaches
- muscle aches
- upset stomach

Dr. Thea Gallagher observes that people are now more productive than they were before the COVID-19 pandemic, that they're working hard and trying to do their best. "But now we're seeing huge levels of burnout—highest numbers we've ever seen. During this time it's easier for people to write an angry email or express a complaint than to say, 'thank you.' People are feeling like 'I did a good job, but I can't do it anymore.'" She notes that people feel like they're robots or on an assembly line, like they're not being acknowledged, not connecting, maybe eating lunch alone, constantly saying "I'm putting out fires everywhere," and feeling distressed.

Author interview with Dr. Thea Gallagher, January 15, 2021

- poor self-care (hygiene)
- fatigue, exhaustion, or feeling overwhelmed
- lack of energy, being stretched too thin
- difficulty sleeping (insomnia)

Protect against Burnout

How do you protect against burnout and keep from losing yourself? The best way is to pace yourself and take time for self-care. Paying attention to your own needs does not mean you are ignoring your responsibilities, work, or your loved ones' needs. Instead, it enables you to be a more available and effective parent, caregiver of senior parents, and coworker.

Doing your best to care for yourself physically, mentally, and emotionally means trying to get sufficient and regular sleep, exercise, and relaxation, as well as ensuring a balanced diet and nutrition plan (as outlined in chapter 9). Keep a steady and consistent sleep schedule and aim to get some physical exercise on most days of the week. Try to keep up with your own friends and support people, those who sustain you, and see them regularly— don't brush them aside for your other duties. Open sharing of your concerns, struggles, and fears with a nonjudgmental person can help facilitate social support.

Lack of control in our lives can contribute to burnout. We need to understand and accept the difference between what we can control, what we may be able to somewhat influence, and what is out of our control. We also need to understand and deal with the traits many of us have that may contribute to feelings of burnout, such as striving for perfection; being highly self-critical; working long hours; working in a high-demand, low-resource setting; putting others' needs first; delaying our self-care; hiding our struggles; and not asking for help.

A shift to taking charge of our own lives again can help in preventing burnout. This includes reexamining and simplifying

our work and home life and our social relationships; setting realistic expectations for what and how much we're willing to take
on and communicating those to others; creating reasonable and
clear boundaries or ground rules; limiting our time spent online
and in nonessential activities; and asking for support.

Specifically, this means we aim to work fewer hours with less
overtime; strive for a balance in work and personal or family
life; learn and use effective coping skills; seek out social connections and support; use relaxation strategies; follow healthy lifestyle behaviors in diet, sleep, exercise, pleasurable activities, and
so forth; and monitor ourselves for warning signs and personal
triggers of burnout. It's also helpful to avoid thinking in *should*
statements ("I should do ____"). These generally reflect unrealistic expectations that can never be met. Instead, say something
like "I'd like it if I had more ____ with my ____."

Do your best to manage life's little daily stressors before they
explode into unmanageable problems. You might break large

*Pace yourself. Do what you
can do now and don't feel
guilty about it.*

tasks into smaller projects, prioritize
the demands placed on you, and learn
to say "no" on occasion. Saying no is
hard for many of us, so you have to
remind yourself that you cannot help your loved ones if you are
stretched too thin.

Do your best to keep your usual routine and maintain structure in your life. Make it a priority in your daily calendar. Look
to your own needs and wants, doing what increases your own
self-esteem and pleasure (hobbies, interests, skills, or volunteer
work). These are what make your life rewarding and rich, what
sustain you. If you're working from home or in a job search,
create a workday routine as if you're at your usual workplace:
get up at the same time; get nicely dressed; or "pretend commute" by walking around the block before you start work. Make
it a point to take mini-breaks throughout the day to clear your

head and restore your energy. Last, treat yourself to something special every once in a while—a meal out, a bouquet of flowers, a new book to read—and don't feel guilty doing so. Many find it refreshing to take time for some activities that bring them pleasure.

Restoring control of our lives may also include working with our employers to address the cultural work environment, procedures, or conventions that can lead to burnout. For example, you may need to both agree that you will not be responding to email messages at night and during off-work hours.

Some people find brief supportive psychotherapy helpful at these times. It may help us understand and recognize the warning signs and personal triggers that could lead to burnout. Therapy could be individual, or it might include joining a support group specifically for friends and families of those who have depression. You can find these groups within the National Alliance on Mental Illness (NAMI) and the Depression and Bipolar Support Alliance (DBSA), national organizations with local chapters that have small groups specifically for family members of those who have a mood disorder. In these groups, you can speak with others like yourself who find themselves in a similar situation with similar problems and share coping strategies.

CHAPTER 5

The Ability to Grieve

BEREAVEMENT, GRIEF, AND PROLONGED GRIEF RESPONSE

Social isolation and the COVID-19 pandemic may affect our ability to bereave and grieve the major life losses we encounter. Bereavement is the experience of losing someone or something you love, and grief is the natural psychological reaction to that loss. This experience is shared by all persons and across every culture. Grief is a strong and sometimes overwhelming emotion, a collection of thoughts and responses related to loss, with yearning and pangs of sorrow, loneliness, and sometimes emptiness. It can result from any type of loss—the loss of a loved one, a relationship, a job, a home, financial security, our sense of personal safety, social connections, normal routines, personal freedoms, our sense of who we are, our self-esteem, or our purpose. For example, if you think of yourself as part of a couple or as having a certain job, loss of these may likely affect your self-image and confidence.

Social isolation adds to our sense of loss and affects our ability to grieve those losses, as does living through an infectious disease outbreak such as the COVID-19 pandemic or having a mental illness. We grieve the loss of our familiar lives and communities as we know them, including personal finances, jobs, opportunities, changes in our world, lifestyle, work, school, home life, health, and well-being in ourselves and loved ones. We grieve the loss of loved ones to a COVID-19 infection. Dr. Thea Gallagher, a clinical psychologist at the University of Pennsylvania, reminds us that during the COVID pandemic, we've had a state of grief almost constantly because there has been much change in our lives, and with every change comes some kind of loss. And a few people may delay or avoid the grieving process for certain losses because they think they can handle only so much emotional distress.

During periods of social isolation or a pandemic we may grieve the illness and loss of life of someone close to us. The death of a loved one may be sudden and unexpected, and often happens alone or amid caring strangers. We now face having to care for them and grieve in a different way, without being able to be there, hold their hand, assist and attend to them when ill or in their final hours of life, or to plan and participate in the funeral or burial rituals customary for our culture. Our likelihood of experiencing grief is increased when we see our loved one in pain; the loss was sudden and unexpected; we cannot say good-bye to them; a death occurred in a hospital; a death was preventable; and if end-of-life treatments were invasive or against the person's wishes. All this may lead us to feel guilt or anger.

Give yourself—and your child—permission to feel sad, depressed, anxious, frustrated, or angry and to grieve.

Normally we participate in certain practices and traditions after a loved one dies that bring us support and closure. Funerals, wakes, shivas, and memorial celebrations of life can often ease the pain of the loss. These are symbolic events that are a really important part of the human experience, giving us time to grieve our loved ones and process the loss. Amid social isolation or the pandemic, however, the routines and rituals that normally bring us comfort, support, healing, and closure aren't readily available. We're left to painfully feel the emptiness and loss when dealing with their estate issues, outstanding bills, and tasks previously done by them. Experiencing the death of a loved one in this way adds to our feelings of isolation and loss, affects our mental health, and can lead to depression, anxiety, PTSD, and prolonged grief disorder.

In addition, when isolated socially, we may also find ourselves grieving the loss of our prior coping strategies and traditions, such as sharing a meal with friends, going to the gym or a barbecue, and so on. We may experience less social support and a greater sense of loneliness. Without the use of the familiar coping strategies we've come to rely on for years, it's likely more difficult to get through these rough times.

Last, having a mental illness often leads to many other life losses and disappointments—some temporary, some prolonged. These include a loss of hopes, dreams, opportunities, employment or career, finances, housing, relationships, perceived social standing, time, self-esteem, and self-respect. We must grieve these losses just as we would any other type of loss. That can be difficult because having a mental illness often affects our ability to grieve. Here's an example:

> *In my conversation with Dr. Douglas Katz, we focused on the difficulties people have in experiencing grief and bereavement during the COVID-19 pandemic, particularly someone who has a mental health disorder such as depression or bipolar disorder. He has observed previously functioning people, whose prior mental illness had been stable, now struggle when a loved one contracts the viral illness and then passes away. The situation is made worse by the person not being able to speak or be with their loved one during the COVID illness or at the moment they pass. While this is devastating to all persons, the individual who has a prior mental health condition may withdraw in response and experience a setback in their illness.*
>
> *Dr. Katz points out that grief is a very interpersonal process. When we're able to grieve in connection with others who were close to the person who was lost, it seems to go much more*

smoothly. There is support that carries the person through this loss. If unable to grieve with others, people can feel lost or stuck, with a sense of not moving on in life because it doesn't feel like much has been resolved.

Dr. Katz has seen people in this situation become fearful of what will happen when the pandemic ends—they worry if there will be fresh waves of grief when they get back in touch with extended family members. They're also concerned about slipping back into a very deep episode of depression at that point.

Author interview with Dr. Douglas Katz, December 28, 2020

Our Response to Loss and Bereavement

In response to any loss, we may go through different stages of grief and mourning, in varying degrees and order based on the individual. We may feel numb or empty, angry, unable to feel joy or sadness; have trouble sleeping or eating; experience excess fatigue, shakiness, muscle weakness, or nightmares; or withdraw socially. Many feel a loss of normalcy and daily routine, of intimate and social connections, of safety, financial security, opportunities, employment, or home environment. In our grief we often mourn the loss of our past way of life and experience anxiety in anticipation of an uncertain future.

Common reactions to grief have been grouped into five *stages* first described by Elisabeth Kübler-Ross in her 1969 book *On Death and Dying*—these are still accepted today. They are:

- Denial and isolation—fear, shock, numbness, disbelief, avoidance of thinking about the loss
- Anger—often with frustration and anxiety, sometimes directed toward a health care provider
- Bargaining—these are "If only" statements or attempts to make a secret deal with a higher power

- Depression—emotional distress, sadness, feeling over-whelmed and helpless
- Acceptance—coming to terms with the loss, marked by a sense of calm (not everyone reaches this stage)

We do not all experience these stages of grief in the same order, time frame, or manner—grief is different for each person and does not progress in a straight line. Often our emotions fluctuate, ranging from moments of sadness, mourning, anger, guilt, to acceptance or sometimes positive feelings about the future and its possibilities. For most, grief subsides over time, and despite it changing our world, we're able to bounce back and move on with our lives. We're able to find ways to normally accept and adapt to our loss and restore a sense of purpose, meaning, and possibilities for happiness. But for others, grief remains persistent, with emotional distress and impaired functioning. This is called *prolonged grief.*

Prolonged grief disorder is a persistent and pervasive yearning, longing, or preoccupation with thoughts and memories of the loss. This grief-related emotional pain causes significant distress and impairment in function that can last six months or longer and exceed our normal cultural customs.

Sometimes the thoughts, feelings, and behaviors we have can interrupt the grieving process, leading to prolonged grief disorder, such as

- viewing the future as empty and meaningless
- excessively avoiding reminders of the loss
- having problems accepting the loss
- being socially isolated and withdrawn
- experiencing survivor guilt

It's been estimated that prolonged grief disorder occurs in about 10 percent of bereaved persons. The COVID-19 pandemic, however, is a time of collective sorrow and has increased the number of persons experiencing grief and prolonged grief. Several million people worldwide are grieving the loss of an estimated 4.95 million loved ones to COVID; the numbers are higher if we include those experiencing the loss of people in their broader social network.

Many people living in social isolation during the COVID-19 pandemic have experienced one or several losses they perceive as smaller or less significant in comparison to the death of a loved one—they believe that others have it much worse than they do. For example, a person might experience the loss of milestones and occasions like graduations, weddings, and proms; time with family and friends; opportunities; and jobs. These moments are what add flavor to our lives. Yet these losses might not be considered important because they're not life threatening. Some of us fail to acknowledge these losses as significant to our lives and mental health and thus do not take the time to grieve them.

Try to remember that your feelings are real and valid, and if you have a loss, *any* loss, you will need to grieve it. Tell yourself that it's okay to feel as you do and give yourself permission to mourn or grieve your loss. If you do not adequately address and reconcile with your loss, it most certainly will come back to haunt you at the most inconvenient times.

COPING WITH GRIEF

Many people have found benefit and relief in following certain coping strategies after a loss; these are listed below. One note regarding the loss of a loved one: there are some actions you can take before the fact that may help you with grief-related stressors, such as talking with your loved one about advanced care planning; specifying each person's preferences for funeral arrangements; or arranging for compassionate care or hospice from providers as needed.

Here are some suggestions for ways to manage your grief:
- Identify and acknowledge the loss.
- Spend some time thinking about the loss and what it means to you, how it affects you, and process those thoughts. Sit with them. Allow yourself to feel your feelings, to feel the grief, anger, and despair. But don't be obsessive about it or let it consume you.
- Accept and come to terms with the loss, that it happened, the reality and finality of the loss and its consequences.
- Focus and rely on your strengths and coping skills.
- If you have lost a loved one, create an end-of-life ritual for them, even if done virtually for now, that will bring you comfort, support from others, and closure.
- Create or do something that honors your loss, a warm and positive reminder of your loved one, such as a memory book, an activity, or planting a tree.
- Find ways to express your grief from other losses, perhaps through art, music, gardening, volunteering, or whatever form of expression you prefer.
- Stay connected. Seek out spiritual support and social support from friends, family, or support groups. Pursue grief counseling with a therapist as needed. Create new rituals in your day to stay in touch with loved ones.
- Take care of yourself. Practice calming and coping strategies and maintain daily routines.

Take these steps to process your loss, come to terms with it, and put it to rest in a corner of your mind, then keep going on with your life. Most people are able to bounce back. They find ways to accept and adapt to their loss, restoring their sense of purpose, meaning, and possibilities for happiness. There is a sense of control in acceptance, a sense of belonging and strengthening of ongoing relationships. Adapting to loss means having a focus on the present, controlling what we can, and letting go of what we can't. It means seeing the future as holding possibilities for a life with purpose and meaning, joy and satisfaction.

And although your loss may pop up in your mind periodically, if you have adequately dealt with it, these intrusive thoughts will remain small and not be disabling. Otherwise, if you do not deal with your loss, if you try to ignore it or push it aside, then painful thoughts and memories will periodically disturb you and interfere with the quality of your life.

When my mom was alive, she was "in charge" of the geraniums, and since her passing, I've made sure to always have a potted red geranium in her memory.

HELPING YOUR KIDS GRIEVE

Many are wondering how we can help our children through the uncertainty and grief of social isolation and the pandemic. Children and adolescents experience grief in a different way than adults. Sometimes children appear sad or may change their behavior by acting out, being irritable, showing disinterest in usual activities, or experiencing changes in their sleep and eating habits. Their grief may interfere with schoolwork or relationships with friends and family. Other times they may be silent about their grief and appear to continue in their usual activities. Adolescents may become more isolated and withdrawn, appear irritable or frustrated, experience changes in sleep and eating patterns, or spend more time using technology.

What can parents do? You as parents can help your children process their grief. Respect your kids' feelings and acknowledge them as valid. We all process and express our feelings in different ways, and their perception of loss will vary by age, gender, personality, and the circumstances. Allow yourself and your children the space to feel your feelings. Ask questions so that you will know what's going on within them and provide age-appropriate answers to their questions. Encourage your children to talk or express their thoughts and emotions in other creative ways—drawing, creating small plays or shows, listening to or creating music, and so forth. This gives them permission to grieve. Teach your children calming and coping strategies and practice these strategies with them. Maintain usual school, family, and social routines as much as possible, even if there are new routines because of the COVID-19 pandemic—children rely heavily on routine and structure. Spend time reading together, coloring, or doing other activities they enjoy. And don't forget to take care of yourself; this is how you role model healthy self-care and coping strategies for your child.

In addition to the above, a recent *Washington Post* article (Koh 2021) has some other interesting suggestions that Dr. Wendy Silverman of the Yale Child Study Center agrees are often helpful. In kids, try to pair an activity with stress release. Engage in different kinds of activities, outside your routine or ordinary tasks, as a way to express isolation or COVID-related emotions. Put the video games and Zoom aside, both kids and parents, and find other ways to connect with friends and family, including having your kids play outdoors with their friends (with masks as appropriate). It's also important to embrace our familiar rituals—purposeful, meaningful practices that bring us comfort. This might be as simple as having dinner together and a family conversation. Rituals help us bond and safely process what's going on. Last, try to identify and include small, simple "low-bar" comforts in your day, like setting up the coffeemaker ahead of time so it will be ready to go in the morning. Caring for yourself in this way will help keep you calm and steady, demonstrating that you matter; when your children observe this, they will learn effective strategies to soothe themselves.

Dr. Silverman believes that the key to dealing with social isolation and the pandemic with your children is "talking through with your child, communicating, and sharing with them what the concerns are and trying to talk it through." She cautions that "at some point it might be too much for the parents to handle . . . that there's only so much reasoning that works." This is particularly true for those children and adolescents who experience preexisting anxiety symptoms. For them, she believes that "reassurance is sometimes the worst thing you can do for these kids because then it becomes a vicious cycle." Anxious children continually want reassurance—having the parent provide it endlessly only reinforces that cycle. It's difficult for parents, so the Yale Child Study Center has developed strategies to help parents learn how to stop the *reassurance-seeking cycle*, things like the parent saying, "Look, I'm going to respond to your question *one* time, and that's all." If that initial approach fails, Dr. Silverman says that "the child might need the more professional approach. The parents need help in learning how to stop the reassurance, and the kid needs to get help to learn how to stop the reassurance seeking by learning their own coping skills" (Silverman interview).

Teens and Young Adults

Teens and young adults are experiencing many losses at this time in addition to the potential loss of a loved one, including missing school and work routines, hanging out with friends, social events and parties, proms, sporting events, or graduation. They may be frustrated, angry, or resentful. Your first step is to recognize that your children may be grieving these losses. Find out what their friends are doing to manage during social isolation or the pandemic, and what things you could do to help your children through this time. Supportive and creative time with family and close friends is one strategy to deal with social isolation, but it's not enough to just increase your children's social contacts. Find ways to help your kids identify alternatives that are meaningful and valid to them, and to help them build structure and purpose in their current lives. Help them connect, balance family and alone time, and find ways to cope with the change and loss. Seek professional help if you think your child is not doing well emotionally or is experiencing loneliness or a mental illness like depression or anxiety, as described in chapters 2 and 6.

CHAPTER 6

Isolation and Mental Health

In this chapter I review several of the more common mental health conditions brought on or affected by social isolation. These include anxiety, depression, post-traumatic stress disorder (PTSD), and post-traumatic growth (PTG). I then discuss how to manage your mental illness and the effects of stigma.

ANXIETY

Anxiety is a feeling of excessive worry, apprehension, and nervousness about future events or activities. The depth of the anxiety or worry, length of time it lasts, and how often it occurs is out of proportion to the actual feared event and causes emotional distress. The fear seems very real and scary to us at the time. It's difficult to control our feelings of worry when we're anxious, and the anxiety is often accompanied by other psychological or vague physical symptoms, such as feeling restless, shaky, or irritable, with difficulty concentrating and disturbed sleep. You may feel nervous, jittery, worried, and sweaty, with your heart racing or skipping a beat. You may have a headache, an upset stomach, and muscle aches. Some people are frightened by these symptoms and go to the Emergency Department, convinced that something is wrong with them physically.

Experts have identified several types of anxiety; here I focus on generalized anxiety disorder, social anxiety, and separation anxiety.

> Dr. Wendy Silverman points out that "the core of anxiety is in not being able to predict and not being able to control . . . and the more that people feel that they cannot predict and they cannot control, the more difficult it is. And so the changes [coming from] . . . everything about COVID, the whole change [in our lives] and the uncertainty, and the fact that it just kind of came [on us suddenly] was really, really difficult. If you're prone to anxiety in the first place, it's certainly going to make it even more challenging for you."
>
> Author interview with Dr. Wendy Silverman, January 14, 2021

Generalized anxiety disorder (GAD) is a term used to describe persistent and excessive worry, more than what you might expect for a given event. A person may assume the worst outcomes even when there is no apparent reason for concern. Anxiety affects about 6.8 million adults in the United States and may be related to biological factors, family background, and stressful life experiences. Approximately half of those who have depression experience anxiety at the same time (Fava et al. 2004; Regier et al. 1998). This adds a great burden to the weight of feeling distressed.

The fifth edition of the *Diagnostic and Statistical Manual of Mental Disorders (DSM-5)*, which is the standard manual used by providers in identifying mental illness, lists criteria for generalized anxiety disorder; these are shown in table 6.1. The *DSM-5* specifies that for a GAD diagnosis, the anxiety must involve various events and activities in combination, such as work, school, and social performance. The individual must find it difficult to control the worry. The anxiety, worry, or physical symptoms must cause significant distress in social, occupational, academic, or other areas of functioning. In addition, the disturbance must not be due to substance use (e.g., drug abuse), medications, or

TABLE 6.1 Criteria for Generalized Anxiety Disorder

To make a diagnosis of generalized anxiety disorder, a person's anxiety and worry must be associated with three or more of the following symptoms, occurring on more days than not for at least six months:

- restlessness, or feeling keyed up or on edge
- being easily fatigued
- difficulty concentrating; mind going blank
- irritability
- muscle tension
- sleep disturbance

Source: American Psychiatric Association, *Diagnostic and Statistical Manual of Mental Disorders*, 5th ed. (Washington, DC: APA, 2013).

another medical condition and is not better explained by another mental disorder.

As adults we tend to worry about common everyday events such as our jobs, finances, our health, the health and safety of our family members, and minor matters (doing household chores or being late for an appointment). It's thought that those of us who have generalized anxiety overestimate the level of danger in these areas and in our surrounding environment, struggle with uncertainty in our lives, and underestimate our own capacity to cope. Anxiety symptoms often occur in those affected by social isolation or an infectious disease outbreak. We fear becoming infected with the virus; fear for our future livelihood and providing for our families; and have other fears. Anxiety can lead to *hypervigilance*, which is when we're constantly on the lookout for bad things to happen, and to *avoidance* of certain situations like certain places or social interactions. Many of us are able to view our situation realistically and can manage the anxiety, while others find it disabling.

Anxiety is the most common form of psychiatric illness in children. The combination of depression and anxiety is common, seen in more than one-half of children who experience anxiety, and it can lead to a more difficult diagnostic assessment, more severe symptoms, and more complicated treatments. These children and adolescents may be reluctant to attend school, play, and interact with others for fear of being evaluated and judged by others or of feeling humiliated or embarrassed in public by some perceived misstep. Kids can be hard on each other, which compounds a child's anxiety. Your child may have increased bodily complaints of physical illness (stomachaches, for example, with missed days of school); irritability and agitation; impaired academic and social functioning during their important developmental years; obsessive thoughts and compulsive behaviors; and increased risk of suicide.

Adolescents tend to worry excessively about their competence, appearance, fitting in socially, schoolwork, sports performance, catastrophic events (nuclear war, terrorism), or their future. As in adults with anxiety, these worries are excessive, interfere with their functioning, and are of long duration and more distressing than the normal worries of everyday life.

Treating anxiety and depression in adolescence is important because early onset of these conditions increases the risk of depression in adulthood. Early intervention in depression and anxiety in adolescence may decrease the burden of illness in later life.

Another type of anxiety, *social anxiety*, is an intense and excessive fear of being judged, humiliated, or rejected in a social situation or being embarrassed in a public performance (giving a speech, playing sports, dancing, or playing a musical instrument on stage). A person is often self-conscious in front of others and may fear stumbling over words, making a mistake, or being viewed as stupid, clumsy, boring, or incompetent. Many of us who experience social anxiety also have physical symptoms, such as a racing heart rate, nausea, and sweating. Anxiety symptoms may be so extreme and disruptive to daily life that they interfere with our routines, school or job performance, or social life, making it difficult to complete school; interview for, get, and hold down a job; and have friendships and romantic relationships—anything that requires interaction with new people. As a result, some people avoid social or performance situations completely, and when these situations can't be avoided, they experience significant anxiety and distress.

My dreaded first attempt at public speaking as a teenager was notable for anxiety, with a dry mouth, sweaty palms, butterflies in my stomach, and verbally mixing or twisting my words in front of everybody—something we called "mush mouth."

Dr. Wendy Silverman has observed quite a bit of variation in how kids react to the isolation of the pandemic. Their reactions seem to be related to the type of underlying problems they have. Take, for example, social anxiety. "These are kids who typically have a hard time going and doing things involving other people out of the fear and anxiety of social evaluation and humiliation. And they stay away from these things, whether it be peer functions, other things. Maybe they go to school, but if they do, it's really hard for them to speak in the class or talk to the teacher or go to the bathroom.

"But interestingly, because they're at home [during the pandemic], those problems are not arising. [COVID-19 has prevented them] from going out and practicing skills and doing things." She explains that, when we do behavioral therapy, it typically helps children gradually face the things that make them anxious by exposing them to it in small steps. Therapists also help the parents learn how to not accommodate anxiety and how to help their child not avoid anxiety-provoking situations. But now, during COVID-19, that's not happening.

(continued)

"*In children, social isolation and the COVID pandemic rep-
resent a change for them. Whatever adaptations they've made,
whether they have a problem that brings them to treatment
or not, there's now a change. There is a different way of going
to school, relating to friends, relating to family members. And
that's particularly disruptive for many, particularly those who
find safety in standardization and in knowing what to expect
from their time. And so some might unravel with just the concept of change.*"

"*For some of the kids, it's like, 'Oh, yeah. Keep this COVID
thing going a long time.' They like not having to do their behavioral therapy and face their anxiety and fears. But for other
kids, while some of the social things they're able to avoid, other
things are really, really hard and stressful. It's like 'I don't want
to do the Zoom.' For some, Zoom is even more scary than meeting people, even though meeting people in public is part of social
anxiety for some kids. [That's because] a Zoom experience is self-
focused attention, which is an element of anxiety. When you're
speaking in front of a group, you mainly have to focus on being
scared and worrying about everybody else. But now you have to
worry about how you look on Zoom, which can be really hard
for people when they're so concerned not about just what other
people think, but also what they think about themselves. So, it's
almost a double whammy.*"

*Dr. Silverman wonders what's going to happen when this
period of isolation is over—she believes it's a really interesting,
intriguing, unclear situation.*

Author interview with Dr. Wendy Silverman, January 14, 2021

Separation anxiety occurs when someone forms a strong
attachment to a person or a thing and reacts strongly to separation from that attachment—parents, caretakers, or things they
are tied to (beyond the infancy stage, when it's normal). It may
be seen in adults or children who "just can't let go." Separation

anxiety can become a problem when it interferes with ordinary activities and normal childhood or adolescent development.

One example of this is seen in children and adults who are compulsively attached to their digital devices, texting, gaming, and social media. These are all designed to be addictive, and the thought of disconnecting from them is unbearable to the person. Normally, our self-esteem and self-worth come from our achievements and real-life personal successes. But, for example, if a person is strongly attached to their electronic devices, they instead rely artificially on the number of "followers" or "likes" they have on social media. Excess reliance on technology restricts real-life activities and sets up a vicious cycle of anxiety, withdrawal, isolation, depression, and fear of separation from the device.

Some of the signs of excessive digital use include:
• using digital media as an escape from emotional discomfort or depressed mood
• isolation or withdrawal from in-person contact with friends and family
• being unable to stop the use of digital devices

Anxiety is a treatable condition. Many therapies and strategies used for depression are also effective options for treating anxiety, such as certain medications, talk therapy, relaxation exercises, and mindfulness meditation. CBT, or cognitive behavioral therapy, can help people restructure their thoughts to understand that their worry is not productive and can teach them relaxation skills. Treatment can help people balance their fears and sense of danger in the world, deal with uncertainty, and learn effective coping skills. In addition, lifestyle changes can reduce their symptoms, such as improving the quality and duration of sleep, getting regular physical exercise (e.g., aerobics and yoga), minimizing caffeine and alcohol use, and avoiding nicotine (tobacco) and street drugs—even during a pandemic.

Exposure therapy is also sometimes used for anxiety as a way to break the deep patterns of fear and avoidance.

DEPRESSION

Normally, we experience moods that change over time and across a broad range of emotions. We can feel happy, sad, irritable, agitated, and many other moods. Most people can feel a bit low and sad at times—normal reactions to life's ups and downs and stressors. Losing a loved one, getting fired or divorced, living in isolation or through the life changes of a pandemic, and other difficult situations can lead a person to feel sad, lonely, and afraid. Some of us, however, experience deeper, more intense symptoms that tend to persist longer, leading to depression.

Depression, also called major depression, major depressive disorder, or unipolar depression, involves our state of mind— the part of our inner self that colors and drives our thoughts, feelings, and behaviors. It's a biologically based, treatable mental health condition of the mind and body that affects our thoughts, feelings, behaviors, relationships, activities, interests, and many other aspects of life. When we're depressed, our mood is persistently very down, and our mental and physical functioning is not as sharp as usual. We don't think as clearly, organize ourselves, or do things as well as before. Someone who experiences depression often has trouble functioning in the ordinary activities of daily living and has an impaired quality of life. These are symptoms of the illness and are not intentional or signs of laziness.

Major depression is closely related to the symptoms and experience of depression seen in bipolar disorder, known as *bipolar depression*. Bipolar disorder is characterized by periodic episodes of extreme elevated mood or irritability, called *manic* or *hypomanic episodes*, alternating with episodes of extreme depression, or *bipolar depression*. These episodes come in cycles;

the pattern differs for each person, although there are usually more episodes of depression.

With any depression, a dark, negative mood may creep up on us silently, or it may be related to external or internal events in our lives. *External events* are things that happen to us or around us. A job loss, a relationship breakup, a visit with a controlling parent, and living in isolation or through a pandemic are examples of negative external events. *Internal events* are the thoughts and feelings inside us, like believing we are unlovable or undesirable. External and internal events can act as triggers to cause a change in our mood. *Triggers* are events or circumstances that may cause a person distress and increase their depression symptoms—they are unique to each person.

The most common symptoms of depression are listed in table 2.2, from the *DSM-5*. To be diagnosed with major depression, you must have at least five of these symptoms, lasting for two weeks or more (and at least one of the symptoms must be persistent sadness or loss of interest). People can have many different combinations of these nine *DSM-5* criteria for depression.

TABLE 6.2 Criteria for Depression

- Sad, depressed, or irritable feelings most of the day
- Loss of interest or pleasure in most activities
- Sleep changes—too much, too little, or with early morning awakening
- Weight loss or gain (without trying)
- Loss of energy
- Decreased ability to think or concentrate
- Restlessness or the sensation of being physically slowed down
- Thoughts of worthlessness, hopelessness, guilt
- Thoughts of death and suicide

Source: American Psychiatric Association, *Diagnostic and Statistical Manual of Mental Disorders*, 5th ed. (Washington, DC: APA, 2013).

Symptoms of depression may differ in women, men, and adolescents. It's important to recognize these differences and direct treatment to their specific symptoms. Women may commonly experience sadness, tearfulness, trouble with sleep, appetite, and fatigue, and may have mood shifts related to their reproductive hormone cycles, pregnancy or the postpartum period, or menopause. Men may demonstrate greater irritability and agitation, become workaholics, drink to excess or abuse substances. Adolescents may appear withdrawn, irritable, anxious, lose interest in school or sports, and have a decline in school grades. All of these are depression.

While a person may experience depressive symptoms related to the stressors and losses of social isolation or the COVID-19 pandemic right now, depression is most often a relapsing and remitting yet treatable illness. *Relapsing and remitting* means that the symptoms come and go, in varying intervals of time called *episodes*. An episode of depression may last weeks, months, or longer. It may differ in how deep or severe it is. Many people

> *Dr. Wendy Silverman believes that symptoms of irritability are a problem and that she is seeing more of it. In her experience "irritability is sort of like having a fever" in that it's a common sign that cuts across many illnesses and diseases, particularly across anxiety and depression. She's observed her patients "showing a lot of irritability, of being touchy and easy to get angry, and as the parents describe them, 'you have to walk on eggshells.'" Dr. Silverman notes that irritability is a predictor of not doing as well in traditional anxiety treatment. She concludes that we are probably addressing it more than we used to in the past, not just how to manage anxiety, but also strategies to help parents manage their children's irritability.*

Author interview with Dr. Wendy Silverman. January 14, 2021

have repeat episodes over time and feel well in between—the pattern is unique to each person. Some have one or a few episodes and then none for many years. It's nearly impossible to predict the duration of each episode and to know exactly if or when a person may have future episodes. It's important to know this because you can take steps now to minimize or eliminate the chance of a recurrence.

What Causes Depression?

The brain is a network of brain cells (called *neurons*) bathed in special chemicals (*neurotransmitters*) that help the cells communicate with each other, sending messages from cell to cell. One long-held theory of depression is that it involves a disruption of these neurotransmitters, which are found throughout the brain, including in the part that regulates our emotions and behavior. The chemical disruption may happen when certain life experiences occur in a susceptible person.

A more recent theory of depression is that the interaction of our genes with events in our lives (our environment) shapes the complex network of cells in our brain. This is called the *gene × environment* theory. Our *environment* includes the people, thoughts, and events that occur around us, both inside and outside our bodies. This could be inside or outside stress, an illness such as COVID-19 in self or loved ones, or a traumatic event, including being in isolation or living through the coronavirus pandemic. Other examples of stressful life events include a major loss or death; being furloughed or losing a job; working from home; balancing work and home education for your children; financial losses; chronic stress; medical illness; substance abuse; and sleep disorders.

A *gene* is a precise arrangement of molecules (a sequence of DNA) that makes up the chromosomes in our cells. Genes are inherited from each of our parents. They direct the body to make certain proteins that control our normal bodily functions, including those of our brain. Scientists have found genes associated with some mental health conditions.

The gene × environment theory of depression is thought to work in this way: The brain is sensitive to stressful and traumatic events during vulnerable periods in our lives. Stress or illness (our environment) changes the action of certain genes. When this happens, it affects the shape of the network of cells in our brain (the *neural network*) and its functioning. If stress or illness changes gene activity during a vulnerable period, the genes and our brains do not work as well. That affects our feelings, thoughts, and behaviors, and the result is depression.

Depression is not entirely genetic and not entirely related to life experiences— it's a combination.

While you may have genetic factors that make you more likely to suffer from depression, this does not guarantee that you will have the illness. If you are genetically prone to depression, you may not have an episode unless you also experience certain stressful life events, such as living through social isolation or a pandemic. These experiences are thought to affect the genes that regulate your brain functioning.

The exciting news is that understanding how genes work in mood disorders will allow researchers to better understand these illnesses and design new treatment interventions. In the future, some of these may be targeted to a person's specific combination of symptoms or subtype of depression (such as seasonal affective disorder; atypical depression; postpartum depression; dysthymia, or persistent depressive disorder; melancholia; etc).

Scientists have also proposed other exciting theories of depression. One cutting-edge theory of depression in 2022 regards mood disorders as an inflammatory process. An illness such as depression would then involve the activation of a cascade of chemical events in the body's immune system. Research scientists are working hard to further our understanding of the inflammatory process and its relationship to mental illness, with the hopes of designing improved and targeted treatments in the future. Stay tuned!

Depression Is a Treatable Illness

Depression is treatable. Possibilities include talk therapy, or psychotherapy; medications, including antidepressants and the newer use of ketamine and esketamine; and neurostimulation treatments, a method that uses either low electrical current (ECT, electroconvulsive therapy, or vagus nerve stimulation) or a magnetic current (rTMS—repetitive transcranial magnetic stimulation) to stimulate the mood centers of the brain. Recent innovations that are also potentially effective include

- identifying and using our specific genes to diagnose a condition and then tailor the optimal dose and type of antidepressant medication to the individual (clinical genomics);
- research on *psychedelic-assisted therapy* for treatment-resistant depression (and other conditions), which increases a sense of well-being and enables a person to work through life issues on a deeper level (different from a conventional treatment approach);
- modifiable lifestyle factors (sleep, diet, exercise, isolation) that impact depression; and
- understanding systemic inflammation as a risk factor for depression.

Many people find that the combination of psychotherapy and medications works the best; it depends on the individual and requires time to try different approaches. More on some of these treatments are presented in chapters 10 and 11.

For a more detailed discussion of depression, see my book *Take Control of Your Depression: Strategies to Help You Feel Better*

Now (Noonan 2018) and Aaron Beck and Brad Alford's *Depression: Causes and Treatment* (2009). There are also many reliable online resources from the National Institute of Mental Health (NIMH) and the Depression and Bipolar Support Alliance (DBSA).

Difficult-to-Treat or Treatment-Resistant Depression

Sometimes, despite trying various medications and treatments, a person may not see improvement in their depression symptoms or level of functioning. Response to treatment often takes weeks or months, and many people require multiple attempts at treatment before they have a satisfactory response. Research has shown that medications are generally helpful in about 60 to 70 percent of people. Only 50 percent of those who have depression respond to a first course of antidepressant treatment, and only 33 percent achieve full remission after a first course (Trivedi et al. 2006). This can all be discouraging for you and your family members.

Currently, psychiatrists see many people who fail to *respond* (defined as partial improvement in symptoms) or to achieve *remission* (defined as complete relief, free of depression symptoms) after an adequate course of treatment. These individuals have what is considered *treatment-resistant depression* (TRD). There is no single definition of or accepted diagnostic criteria for treatment-resistant depression. It may mean failure to improve after one course of an antidepressant of adequate dose and duration, or it may mean failure to respond to three or more courses of antidepressants over several months or more. Historically, the definition of TRD was based solely on medication management and does not align with current clinical practice methods as described above. Factoring in all these other treatments will change the treatment response rates.

Researchers have learned that many factors may contribute to treatment resistance: the medication dosage is too low, the medication was not given for a long enough time and has not been given a chance to work, or the medication is not tolerated well and so the individual has stopped taking it because of side effects. Perhaps it's not the best choice of drug for particular types of symptoms, or the person's diagnosis may not be quite accurate. (For example, it's not uncommon to mistake unipolar depression and bipolar depression at first glance. An episode of elevated mood—mania or hypomania—must be experienced before bipolar disorder can be formally diagnosed. Since that often happens after symptoms of bipolar depression occur, it may lead to delays or unintentional errors in diagnosis.)

Medication options for treatment-resistant depression can be to (1) switch to another antidepressant, (2) augment the antidepressant drug by adding a non-antidepressant drug (such as lithium, atypical antipsychotics, thyroid hormone, herbal products, etc.) to enhance the effects of the antidepressant drug, or (3) combine different types of antidepressants. In addition, we now have new, better-tolerated medications, combined with careful attention to standard psychiatric treatment guidelines by providers, that have improved outcomes.

A replacement term recently proposed for TRD is *difficult-to-treat depression* (DTD). This recommendation is based on the concern that persisting with a series of medication trials that are considered unlikely to achieve remission may be fruitless and pose an undue burden on the patient, not to mention creating unpleasant side effects. DTD is based largely on expert consensus; its purpose is to shift the focus away from a goal of complete remission to one of *optimal symptom control and functional improvement,* where the inconvenience, side effects, and burden of repeated treatments on patients' lives are minimized.

Before declaring that remission is not possible and assigning this new DTD label, the clinician is expected to do a comprehensive evaluation of all treatable causes of the presenting symptoms and confirm the correct diagnosis, adequate treatment (dose and duration), and prior adherence to treatment; consider the pharmacogenetics; and assess general medical and psychiatric *comorbidities* (which are any associated physical or mental health diagnoses) and psychological stressors (environmental factors) that may have

I have often been reminded that in life you never know what is coming around the corner, including treatment possibilities—it's something I hold on to, my reason to be hopeful.

been unrecognized. The goal is then to use all available interventions to evaluate and manage the person's symptoms. Additional treatment options for DTD include psychotherapy and neurostimulation, either ECT or rTMS, to stimulate the mood centers of the brain. The individual would be included in all discussions and decisions in collaborative patient-centered shared decision making. Their illness would be reevaluated periodically, and they would have the right and be encouraged to resume active treatment at a later date as desired.

Even when under the care of experts, some individuals may still be difficult to treat. The DTD model does not mean that the provider has given up hope for the person, or that they will never improve. Its goal is to reduce the burden of illness and treatment efforts on the person. Psychiatrists urge the person who has depression not to despair or give up on treatment. All patients deserve to have hope. My recommendation is to instead modify this line of thinking to one of "the steps to remission are not yet identified for this person" with the view of depression as "treatable with challenges."

The Effect of Depression in Parents on Their Children
Depression, anxiety, and mental health issues in parents, particularly mothers, can lead to mental health and behavioral problems in their children. This is especially true in low-income and

ethnic minority groups; single parents; those with no or inadequate mental health treatment or access to treatment; and those who are reluctant to receive professional mental health care because of concerns related to cost, time, childcare, transportation, cultural issues, stigma, or trust in the system. A consequence of maternal depression is impaired or problematic parenting skills (with negative, disengaged, or withdrawn parenting styles) and being less able to care for her child in an age-appropriate way.

Infants and younger children are more vulnerable because they often have younger mothers who have a higher rate of depression, young children spend more time with mothers during those early years, and these children are undergoing rapid changes in emotional and intellectual (cognitive) development that, following exposure to a parent's depression, have been linked with mental health challenges later in life.

Some children of depressed mothers are found to have decreased cognitive (intellectual) development and a higher risk of mental illness (depression, anxiety) and behavior problems (irritability, hostility, fear). These are not necessarily permanent—interventions can make a difference and can facilitate healthy development.

Interventions for these children include addressing the risk (maternal depression) and the consequences of that risk (poor parenting skills related to having depression). Depression in parents can be treated with cognitive behavioral therapy (CBT), interpersonal therapy, mindfulness-based CBT, medications, and somatic therapies (such as ECT or rTMS—see chapter 10). A combined review of many research studies (called a *meta-analysis*) showed that treatment for depression in mothers was associated with an improvement in their symptoms, improved mental health in their children, better mother-child interactions, and less parenting and marital distress (Cuijpers et al. 2015). Depression treatment alone may not be enough, however, and improved parenting skills are needed (less harsh and critical, more affectionate and smiling, etc.) to achieve better social, emotional, and behavioral outcomes in children. Such improvement would include teaching parents problem-solving, stress and anger management, and communication skills. Examples of effective and cost-effective combined treatments for maternal depression and parenting include home visiting programs, in-home CBT and parenting education, and others.

POST-TRAUMATIC STRESS DISORDER

It's normal to be upset, irritable, and have trouble concentrating and sleeping after we've experienced or witnessed (in person or through the media) a disturbing or traumatic event, especially if it involves a personal assault on our life and well-being. This experience may interfere with our daily activities for a few weeks. But if these symptoms last longer than one to two months, you may have post-traumatic stress disorder (PTSD).

Trauma is considered an emotional response to a distressing event that causes overwhelming stress, exceeding our ability to cope with it. It can provoke fear, helplessness, or horror in response to the threat of injury or death and is a challenge to our sense of safety and vulnerability. Our psychological response to a traumatic event is determined by the features of the event and our own personal characteristics, interpretation of the event, previous trauma experiences, underlying mental health issues, and other factors. It's a perception that varies by our age, gender, stage of life development, and current level of stress and social support. Our reaction to trauma might include feeling nervous or irritable, experiencing unpredictable emotions, having flashbacks, as well as suffering strained relationships, headaches, stomachaches, nausea, rapid heartbeat, or sweating. Trauma can also lead to serious long-term negative mental health consequences such as depression, anxiety, social withdrawal, substance abuse, or PTSD.

PTSD is a severe, disabling mental health disorder, a type of anxiety that sometimes occurs after exposure to a traumatic event. It may develop in those of us who have experienced either an actual or a threatened injury to ourselves or others. For many, the experience of social isolation or living through a pandemic is considered traumatic and can lead to PTSD. Thoughts of being alone in isolation, with little human contact; imposed mandates to follow CDC guidelines and physical restrictions; having limits placed on our personal freedoms and ability to go about in the world—these are negative experiences that may be felt as traumatic. An increased length of time spent in quarantine has also been found to be associated with symptoms of PTSD.

TABLE 6.3 **Criteria for PTSD**

PTSD is defined in the *DSM-5* as a person having

  A. direct or indirect exposure to a threat (death or violence) or serious injury;

  B. reexperience of or reliving the event (unwanted distressing images, memories, nightmares, flashbacks, triggers, emotional distress, or physical symptoms);

  C. avoidance of thoughts, behaviors, events, situations, and places associated with the previous traumatic event;

  D. negative thoughts or feelings; and

  E. feeling keyed up and having increased arousal and activity related to the trauma (irritability; high-risk behaviors; hypervigilance, or being on constant lookout for threats; trouble sleeping or concentrating; being easily startled).

Symptoms must last for more than one month, cause distress or impair the person's functioning, and are not due to medications or substance use.

Source: American Psychiatric Association, *Diagnostic and Statistical Manual of Mental Disorders*, 5th ed. (Washington, DC: APA, 2013).

Symptoms of PTSD can be short (acute) or longer lasting (chronic). They may cause distress at unexpected times, after a trigger, or on the anniversary date of the trauma. *Flashbacks,* which often occur in PTSD, are moments when you feel like you're reliving the traumatic experience again. Memories can return to haunt you at any time, giving you the same fear and horror as the first time. You may also experience *triggers,* which are thoughts, sights, smells, places, situations, or persons—even something on the news—that remind you of the event and cause you to have repeat symptoms.

Hypervigilance, one of the main symptoms of PTSD, is a sense of being constantly on guard and on the lookout for possible traumatic events. *Hyperarousal,* another feature, is an experience of feeling excited, jittery, and keyed up, with trouble sleeping, concentrating, or being excessively startled by certain

> *Dr. Thea Gallagher explains that people who experience PTSD avoid thinking about what happened; they want to avoid any reminders of the event, any connections to the emotions or thoughts associated with it. They believe that the world is unsafe, that they are incompetent and have a shorter lifespan, and that bad things can happen to them at any moment. Yet the more they avoid, the smaller their world gets. That in turn affects their belief in being able to succeed in situations (self-efficacy) and their ability to connect and participate in the world around them.*
>
> *Dr. Gallagher and colleagues at the University of Pennsylvania offer a type of talk therapy for PTSD called prolonged exposure treatment. It's an 8- to 15-session evidence-based treatment proven effective for PTSD based on the idea that people have to experience the emotions associated with the traumatic event, process what they went through, and then get back to living their lives and doing the things they have avoided as a result.*
>
> Author interview with Dr. Thea Gallagher, December 16, 2020

noises. *Avoidance* of thoughts, behaviors, situations, and places associated with the traumatic event, also common in PTSD, reduces our chance to confront our underlying fears surrounding the trauma and reverse them, and prevents us from developing effective coping strategies, resulting in further emotional distress.

Health care workers and first responders who witness serious injury, illness, and death daily are at increased risk for PTSD, as are military veterans following combat experiences. Children may experience PTSD, seen as needing to be close to their parents (under age 6); acting out the trauma in play; nightmares; irritability or aggression; avoiding school; and having trouble with schoolwork or friends. Teens may have symptoms similar to those of adults.

PTSD can be treated with *trauma-focused* psychotherapy, CBT, exposure therapy, and sometimes medications. The VA (Department of Veterans Affairs) and DOD (Department of Defense) have created a thorough clinical treatment guideline for the management of PTSD and acute stress disorder (VA and DOD 2017).

> *Dr. Wendy Silverman has published many studies on the mental health effects of Hurricane Andrew (1992), an example of trauma and isolation, and says that "when we looked at the kids who didn't do well and had persistent reactions of posttraumatic stress, we did find that preexisting anxiety was a risk factor for not doing as well in reaction to the hurricane." Regarding the current COVID pandemic and social isolation and anxiety, she states, "The kids I'm seeing could be more at risk than the other kids in the population in terms of how they're dealing with the COVID [pandemic]."*
>
> Author interview with Dr. Wendy Silverman, January 14, 2021

Post-traumatic Growth

Sometimes a stressful, upsetting, traumatic, or highly challenging experience is followed by positive (psychological) life changes. When this happens, it's called *post-traumatic growth* (PTG). Following such trauma, the person may come to a new belief system or a new understanding of themselves, their world, their future, and how to live their life. They grow in a new direction as a result of the event. The person needs to have an openness and willingness to explore new things in order for this to happen. PTG is not the same as resilience, described in chapter 12.

Psychologists Richard Tedeschi and Lawrence Calhoun (1996) have described five general areas where life changes following trauma can occur:

- improved relationships with others;
- new priorities and decisions giving you new opportunities and life experiences (such as a new job);
- greater appreciation for life;
- an increased sense of personal strength; and
- becoming more spiritual.

HOW TO EFFECTIVELY MANAGE YOUR MENTAL ILLNESS

The best results or outcomes following a mental illness are found in those who learn about the illness and how to manage it, as well as mastering the steps listed below. Your goal will be to manage your illness, reduce the burden of symptoms of anxiety and depression, improve functioning in between mood episodes, prevent recurrence (a return of symptoms), and rely on your resilience—the ability to adapt well in the face of adversity and stress.

How do you do this?

- *Educate yourself about your illness.* Knowledge gives you power and control over your illness. This can be done using reliable information online and in print, with the help of an individual therapist, in family or couples' therapy, or in a psychoeducational support group, presentation, or seminar. When you make the effort to educate yourself about anxiety, depression, grief response, PTSD, and the management of these conditions, the effect will be fewer symptoms, a greater chance of sticking with recommended medications and treatments, a longer time in between repeat episodes, with fewer recurrences over time, and fewer or no inpatient hospital admissions.

• *Illness awareness.* If you have symptoms of a mental illness, become aware that your feelings are symptoms of an illness. Symptoms are not facts; they are not permanent, and they do not define you. Accept having the diagnosis. Also become aware of the symptoms, warning signs, and personal triggers that may signal the worsening course of your depression or anxiety.

• *Stick to treatment.* Taking a medication, attending a weekly support group, or following health-promoting behaviors (getting enough sleep, eating well, exercising) are not too hard to do for a week or two for most of us. The challenge is committing to these activities for a lifetime, accepting the fact that it's sometimes necessary, and keeping yourself motivated. Psychiatric medications and treatments characteristically take several weeks before you see the effects, sometimes up to six to eight weeks, and in that time it's difficult to stick with the treatment regimen, especially when you feel that you're not seeing any positive results yet. This is why it is important to find a mental health provider who is a good fit for you and builds an effective treatment alliance.

• *Detection of early warning signs.* Each person who has depression, anxiety, or PTSD has a characteristic set of signs that signal a change is going on in their emotional health or illness. *Warning signs* are distinct changes from your baseline self that precede a depressive or anxious episode. These changes might be in your thoughts, behaviors, daily routine, or self-care activities. You might notice that you feel less hopeful, more irritable, with a change in your sleep pattern; that you have difficulty with daily household or work routines; or that you've stopped bathing as often. Early recognition of these unique warning signs gives you and your mental health treatment team a chance to intervene and modify (change or improve) the course of the illness. Intervention might include an adjustment in dose, frequency, or type of medication or a different tactic in talk therapy.

- *Lifestyle patterns.* Those who have mental illness are greatly helped by keeping up a regular pattern of healthy lifestyle habits. This includes taking medications as prescribed, following a regular sleep schedule seven days per week, eating healthy food three meals a day, exercising daily, maintaining a structure and routine to your day, and avoiding isolation by keeping up with friends and family members. There is more detailed information on lifestyle patterns in chapter 9.

- Having depression or anxiety does not mean that you'll be unable to manage the stressors of living in social isolation or a pandemic. Focus on maintaining your usual and effective coping and problem-solving strategies, take care of yourself, and pace yourself.

Living with a mental illness is a lot of hard work. We don't know if we'll experience one or more than one episode in our lifetime, but we're much better off if we manage it in ways that reduce its effect on our lives. Managing your mental illness effectively requires that you strive to achieve the following, one or two at a time:

- Accept it as an illness.
- Follow your treatment plan.
- Understand the fluctuations (changes) in your symptoms and the patterns you have.
- Define your baseline.
- Identify and monitor your *triggers*.
- Identify and monitor your *early warning signs* and *symptoms*.
- Develop an *action plan* to use when things get worse, when you or others notice your warning signs.
- Use relapse prevention strategies. Relapse prevention is a day-to-day approach to help you stay well.
- Learn and use effective *coping skills*.
- Maintain social connections. Avoid isolation.
- Maintain self-care.
- Have a daily routine and structure. Schedule your time.
- Do something every day, even when you don't feel like it.
- Build mastery by achieving or improving a challenging skill.
- Develop tolerance for feeling distress for a short time, during a moment of crisis.

For more details on how to manage your illness, I refer you to my book *Take Control of Your Depression: Strategies to Help You Feel Better Now* (Noonan 2018). Along with the above steps, I suggest that you review the treatment options as well as the sections on mindfulness and building resilience found throughout this book.

DEALING WITH STIGMA

In the real world we often have to deal with the effects of the stigma of mental illness, even in the year 2022. A *stigma* is a label or stereotype that is unfairly placed on you by someone without a good, valid reason for doing so. Stigma arises when misinformed people critically judge a person because of some condition, characteristic, or trait, such as being short or having a mental illness, and then unfairly label them with a negative

Comments that arise from the stigma around mental illness are hurtful and untrue.

stereotype or image. Some poorly informed people may believe that it is socially unacceptable to have a mental illness. They may try to make you feel ashamed, humiliated, or disgraced because of the stigma. Others may falsely believe you are incompetent, potentially dangerous, weak in character, or undesirable just because of your illness. They will be harshly judgmental and critical. But they are mistaken.

There is nothing unacceptable about having a biologically based condition such as depression, anxiety, or PTSD (or diabetes or heart disease, for that matter). Unfortunately, many people are not informed about these conditions as illnesses, and they believe in the stigma, the unfair criticism or judgment. They may try to force their inaccurate beliefs and attitudes on you. Ill-informed beliefs and judgments may come from friends, family, or strangers who just don't know any better. These judgments may also come from the media, such as television or social media sites, which tend to sensationalize the news and perpetuate misconceptions. Remember that it's their misinformation driving this behavior.

Stigma can be a barrier to your seeking professional help for mental illness, especially if you fear that others may find out and judge you negatively. Having an illness with a stigma attached is an additional burden to carry on top of the depression or anxiety symptoms you already feel. And having to deal with others' inaccurate reactions to and criticism of your illness can increase your suffering. You may feel that you're constantly choosing whether to feel hurt and deal with that, or face the offender and correct their misinformation, if you have the mental energy to do so.

When others attach a stigma to your illness, it can put a strain on your relationships with them at home, at work, or in social situations. This can result in your being avoided, rejected, or shunned by others. It can lead to an inability to make friends socially because others reject your friendship efforts; a loss of a job or earned promotion for which you're qualified; the loss of housing opportunities; and other unfair actions.

Remaining quiet about one's mental illness to avoid the stigma is not always a good solution, however. Speak up if you are able and the opportunity presents itself, but don't get into an argument. One effective response is for you to step back and understand that you may never be able to turn around the offending person's thinking no matter how hard you try. Aim to consider the source of those distorted beliefs—and try to ignore the comments of those whose opinions you cannot change.

CHAPTER 7

Suicidal Thoughts or Impulses

The most severe form of disturbed emotions, depression, or other mental illness can lead someone to consider self-harm or suicide. Suicide is considered an impulsive act in a troubled person who sees no way to change their painful circumstances. Suicidal thoughts and acts happen when our deep emotional pain or a stressor exceeds our ability to cope with that pain. In the chaos and anguish of the moment, it is often not possible for a person to reach the logical part of their brain to change these troubling and distorted thoughts.

A suicidal act often surprises family members and close friends because the person is not perceived as impulsive and hides their emotional pain deep inside.

Suicide is one of the greatest tragedies in the United States and in the world. In 2020, 45,979 persons committed suicide in the United States (American Foundation for Suicide Prevention [AFSP] 2021b; data from the Centers for Disease Control and Prevention [CDC]). Even before the COVID-19 pandemic, suicide rates were rising in the Unites States, increasing by approximately 25 to 30 percent from 1999 to 2016 in all states but one. Suicide has been the second leading cause of death in those aged 10 to 34, peaking in adolescents, adults, military veterans, and the elderly. It continues as a problem during the COVID-19 pandemic.

Globally, the exact rates of suicide are difficult to obtain. The WHO estimates that 800,000 persons worldwide die from suicide each year. Suicide varies within and between countries. This is partly due to economic conditions and cultural differences, disruption of traditional cultural and family supports, areas of lower socioeconomic status, and increased alcohol and substance use.

The numbers for those who have tried to seriously harm themselves or attempt suicide are also hard to obtain, so they may not be accurate. While many suicide attempts go unreported or untreated, surveys suggest that at least one million people harm themselves each year in the United States.

More than half of those who died by suicide did not have a known diagnosed mental health condition at the time of their death (CDC 2021a). Suicide is not due to any one thing. The CDC report notes that many factors contribute to taking one's life:

- relationship problems or loss
- substance use issues
- physical health problems
- job or financial stress
- recent or impending life crises
- legal problems
- housing stress
- other life stressors

Those without a known mental health condition, according to the CDC report, were more likely to be male or belong to a racial or ethnic minority and less likely to seek help, but anyone struggling with serious lifestyle problems is at risk. Cultural attitudes may also play a part; for example, there is a very high rate of suicide among veterans whose military lifestyle includes a "can do" tough-it-out attitude that often discourages them from seeking help.

One theory that attempts to explain why a person would perform a suicidal act suggests that suicidal behavior involves a vulnerability or predisposition in the person (from a previous trauma or adversity, family genetics, hopelessness, substance use, recent major loss) who then experiences a major stress (acute psychiatric illness, interpersonal problem, life event, social isolation, exposure to or infection with COVID-19, etc.) that triggers the impulsive suicidal act.

Many experts have offered other theories of suicide in an attempt to understand it, yet there is no one model that fits all persons and situations. Some of the ideas that may apply to those living through the COVID-19 pandemic include experiencing:
- hopelessness
- absence of meaningful connections
- inability to cope with problems and losses
- falling short of standards or expectations
- setbacks

In June 2020, during the COVID-19 pandemic, a survey of US adults revealed higher levels of adverse mental health, substance abuse, and suicidal thoughts compared with the time before the pandemic. Among those who responded to the survey, approximately twice as many reported serious thoughts of suicide in the previous 30 days than did adults in the United States in 2018. It was higher in younger adults, racial or ethnic minorities, essential workers, and unpaid adult caregivers (Czeisler et al. 2020).

Some age groups may be more vulnerable to contemplating self-harm or suicide. Many adolescents and teenagers have a difficult time during this phase of their lives. They feel pressure to succeed in school and to fit in with their peers. Most are having a difficult time confined to home during COVID, unable to socialize with their friends, attend school, or play sports. There is added stress in attending school in a hybrid or virtual fashion, where one is unable to interact as usual and cannot read the subtle cues so obvious in direct conversations. Some struggle with self-esteem and self-doubt. This age group also exhibits a fair amount of impulsive behavior. Others may face loneliness, loss of friends or family, and disruption of usual home, work, and social routines. Older adults also experience physical impairments that limit their lifestyle, medical problems and chronic pain, loneliness as family and friends pass on, retirement, or loss of independence and purpose, all of which increases their risk of suicide.

Suicidal thoughts and behaviors of any kind are considered a psychiatric emergency that requires immediate response. If you or your family member shows any signs of suicidal thoughts or intent, call 9-1-1, your PCP or mental health provider, or go to the Emergency Department to get professional mental health evaluation and treatment.

WHAT TO DO

If you feel suicidal, call or sit down with a supportive person and disclose your feelings and thoughts on death and suicide, and any thoughts you may have about harming yourself. Be open and honest about this, and whether you have a plan or the means. If you don't feel comfortable doing this, find someone else to talk to—a minister, teacher or school counselor, your PCP, or a mental health care provider. If you are still uncomfortable, or feel you are in crisis, call 9-1-1 or go to your closest Emergency Department for evaluation and safety.

While thoughts of suicide may seem real and urgent, don't believe them or act on them. Try to recognize that it's the depression driving your thoughts. Our emotions are constantly shifting; they are not permanent or fixed, even if you seem to return to the same familiar ones repeatedly. Although emotions are driven by strong urges, they will change and will pass in time.

One challenge is to get yourself to believe that there are people in your life who love you and are concerned about you.

Your goal is to get through this time safely, until your (temporarily disorganized) mind is able to manage your problems. Once the urgency has passed, you will have time to work on the problems that brought you to this point. Get professional mental health treatment as soon as possible. Suicidal thoughts won't get better on their own without help.

Suicidal thoughts are wayward thoughts, not facts, and will last only a short time. It's hard to wrap your head around that.

If you are concerned about a friend or family member who appears suicidal, sit down with that person and talk. Gently ask questions without judging. Stay neutral and calm. Be supportive and empathetic. Listen with your full attention and encourage them to speak openly about these painful feelings. Be aware that the person may have beliefs and attitudes about suicide that differ from your own (for example, your beliefs that suicide is morally wrong or their beliefs that it's a rational option) and try to separate out your own thoughts and remain neutral.

It can be scary to hear about suicide and to talk about it. If you are unable to have this conversation, call for professional help immediately. If you feel you can speak about it, take a deep breath and stay calm during this conversation. You can be most helpful if you sit and listen to your family member's or friend's thoughts of self-harm and any suicidal thoughts or plans they may have.

Don't underestimate your abilities to help a person who is suicidal. One way to start is to say, "I've been very concerned about you lately. Have you ever thought about harming yourself or wishing that you weren't here?" Let them know you care and that they're not alone. Do your best to listen. You can help by finding out about available resources for people at risk in their area.

Ask them directly and gently if they have specific details or have made a suicide plan: "Do you have a plan?" "What is it?" "When?" and "Do you have what you need to carry out your plan?"

Find out if they are hearing voices and whether the voices are directing them to take action. Know that the lack of a plan does not guarantee their safety. Mental Health First Aid has created a helpful guideline for assessing suicidal thoughts and behaviors, and I have included a link to their page in the list of resources.

Talking with someone about suicide will not cause them to take action.

If your family member shows any indication of suicide intent or a plan, take it seriously. Call for professional help immediately by dialing 9-1-1 or their mental health provider. The goal is to keep your loved one safe and have them evaluated by an experienced mental health professional. In the meantime, remove anything (pills, knives, firearms) from their environment that they might use for this purpose. Do not leave them alone.

Some people fear that speaking of suicide with a person who has depression may make the situation worse. But having this conversation will not encourage them to take action. Asking about suicide and encouraging your family member or friend to get help does not increase the risk of suicide. Rather, it signals to them that you care and gives them an opportunity to talk about their problems. Talking about it may lower the chance of suicide.

Know that while you can offer support and provide for safety, you are *not* responsible for the actions of someone else and cannot control what they might decide to do. It is impossible for even the best-trained mental health professional to accurately predict what actions every person might take, and often these plans are cleverly hidden from others like you.

Also know that the suicidal person may become angry with you and feel betrayed because you interrupted their self-harm plans. Try not to take this personally, including any hurtful words that may come your way. In the long run, speaking up and taking action against suicide is in their best interest. It is better to have them angry with you than to lose them permanently.

SUICIDE PREVENTION AND SAFETY PLANNING

You can take several useful steps in trying to prevent your loved one's suicide. Unfortunately, these are not a guarantee—a person who is strongly committed to suicide may be clever in hiding their intentions and plans and may eventually carry them out despite your best efforts and those of professionals.

First, ensure that they receive a thorough medical and psychiatric evaluation and effective professional care for their mental, physical, or substance use disorders with a combination of medical and mental health treatments. You may want to help them arrange these treatments, since the telephone calls and paperwork required to schedule appointments can be an overwhelming effort for the person. They may also need a referral for these treatments from their primary care physician, depending on their type of health insurance plan.

Second, make sure they have no access to lethal means of suicide: pills, firearms, knives, or other weapons in the home. This means going through the house from top to bottom and removing anything they might be able to use or that might tempt them or put them at risk.

Third, and most important, provide them with support and a strong connection to you, their friends and family, and their community. This includes ongoing support through their medical and mental health providers. A sense of social connectedness can make a big difference. Encourage them to learn and use skills in problem solving, resolving conflicts, and handling their problems in a nonviolent way. In addition, for many people, spiritual and religious beliefs that validate the need for self-preservation and discourage self-harm have been useful.

If you think it can't wait, call 9-1-1 or take them to your local hospital Emergency Department for evaluation. The mental health response team will then decide if and how best to act.

Sometimes having suicidal thoughts or desires means they have to be admitted to the hospital until the crisis passes. That's okay. They will be safe there and evaluated by mental health professionals who will create or modify their mental health treatment plan as needed.

CHAPTER 8

Substance Abuse and Addictions

Some people try to buffer their deep emotional pain associated with a mental illness, social isolation, or COVID-19 by using alcohol, illegal drugs, or other substances. This is especially true if they have newly acquired mental health symptoms and distress that goes untreated. They may not be familiar with treatment options and thus turn to alcohol or other drugs as a way to self-medicate and relieve their painful mental health symptoms. We have seen a rise in this during the social isolation of the COVID-19 pandemic. Substance use may occur occasionally or become a regular problem a person cannot control. It's not an effective strategy, however, and research shows that alcohol and other drugs worsen the symptoms of mental illness.

Some people experience a mental illness and a substance use disorder at the same time—this is called *dual diagnosis.*

> Dr. Thea Gallagher notes that people need to be educated about dealing with their emotional experiences, "that if you don't get help, what we end up seeing is that people, sometimes because they need help, end up doing things like abusing substances" and that "if you leave it neglected you're likely going to end up with more deteriorating symptoms that could impact your life in a greater way."
>
> Author interview with Dr. Thea Gallagher, January 15, 2021

When either of these two conditions occur first—substance use or mental illness—they are referred to as *co-occurring disorders*. According to a 2014 National Survey on Drug Use and Health, 7.9 million people in the United States experienced both a mental disorder and a substance use disorder at the same time (SAMHSA 2014). These numbers have increased during the COVID-19 pandemic.

Substance use and abuse and drug addiction are mental illnesses that change the brain in specific ways.

You might wonder why mental illness and substance use can be linked. Predisposing genetic factors may make a person susceptible to having both addiction and a mental health disorder. In addition, environmental factors in your life—stress, trauma (physical or emotional) and early exposure to drugs—are often overlapping and can influence the development of addiction and other mental illnesses.

The substance most commonly used in excess or abused is alcohol, followed by marijuana (cannabis) and cocaine. Males aged 18 to 44 are at greatest risk. Mental illness and substance abuse are biologically—and physiologically—based and have both mental and physical effects; they are true medical conditions, and the person needs professional help to deal with them. Substance use complicates almost every aspect of care for the person who has a mental illness. It is especially complex and difficult to manage.

Cannabis (marijuana) is the most commonly abused drug in the world, and it has multiple side effects. Among US adolescents, 20.9 percent report use in the past month, and 7 percent of US high school seniors report daily or near-daily cannabis use. The numbers are fairly similar globally. There is known to be an increased and earlier onset of psychosis with cannabis use. *Psychosis* is an altered condition of the mind where the person loses their sense of reality and may have hallucinations, delusions (fixed false beliefs), and disordered thoughts and speech. Psychosis can be caused by some medications, alcohol or drug abuse, or a mental illness, including some forms of depression and schizophrenia.

Scientific studies have confirmed that when cannabis is used in adolescence, the risk of developing depression and suicidal thoughts and behavior in later life increases. Girls seem more likely to develop depression in later life following teenage cannabis use. Side effects include decreased achievement in school, dropping out of school, the potential for addiction, adverse birth outcomes in the offspring of mothers with cannabis habits, and neuropsychological decline with memory loss. Some of this is because the adolescent brain is still developing, and psychotropic drugs may alter the physiologic and neurologic development of the brain.

Substance addiction is a more severe problem than substance use or abuse. Addiction involves regular use in higher amounts than substance use or abuse. In addiction, the person is often unable to stop once using starts, despite the negative consequences or poor health it may cause. Addiction implies physiologic dependence, tolerance, and withdrawal symptoms after stopping drug use.

SYMPTOMS

Someone who has a problem with addiction or dual diagnosis may change their behavior in many ways from their usual self. In addition to the physical influence of the drug, symptoms of substance use or abuse disorder may include:

- withdrawal from friends and family
- sudden changes in behavior
- using substances under dangerous social conditions or settings

- engaging in risky behaviors
- loss of control over use of substances
- developing a high tolerance for the same amount (dose) of the drug
- withdrawal symptoms
- feeling like you need a drug to be able to function

WHAT SHOULD YOU LOOK FOR IN YOURSELF AND OTHERS?

Many people who have a substance use or abuse problem try to hide it from their friends and families in clever ways. Be on the lookout for changes in behavior and physical signs such as:
- sudden financial problems
- failure to meet obligations, such as school or work
- reckless activities (driving while intoxicated)
- legal troubles (getting arrested)
- valuables disappearing from the household
- spending a long time in the bathroom
- dilated or pinpoint pupils
- needle marks on the skin
- drug paraphernalia found in the house (needles, syringes, tourniquets, etc.)

ADDICTION AND ADDICTION TREATMENT

The most effective treatment for dual diagnosis is an *integrated intervention*, when a person receives care for both diagnosed mental illness and substance abuse at the same time. With this treatment, people support each other as they learn about the role alcohol and illegal substances have in their lives. They learn social skills and how to replace substance use with new thoughts and behaviors, as well as receiving concrete help for situations related to their mental illness.

Treatment for dual diagnosis is complex and not easy to do. It is also more expensive. Persons with both mental health and substance abuse conditions have treatment costs that are 61 percent higher, and total medical care costs that are 44 percent higher, than for those who have depression alone.

Stages of Treatment

The treatment process has several stages, and they are not easy. You or your loved one needs to complete each stage and return to treatment as needed if slipups occur.

Detoxification. This is the first stage in which the person stops taking the substance they are abusing and may experience uncomfortable symptoms of withdrawal. Inpatient detoxification is generally more effective than outpatient treatment to achieve initial sobriety and safety. During inpatient detoxification, trained medical staff monitor a person 24/7 for up to seven days. The staff may administer tapering amounts of the substance or its medical alternative to wean a person off and lessen the effects of withdrawal.

Inpatient rehabilitation. Following detoxification, a person experiencing a mental illness and dangerous, dependent patterns of substance use may benefit from an inpatient rehabilitation center, where they can receive medical and mental health care 24/7. These treatment centers provide therapy, support, medication, and health services to treat the substance use disorder and its underlying causes.

Supportive housing. These are residential treatment centers like group homes or sober houses that may help people who are newly sober or trying to avoid relapse. These centers provide some support and independence. Sober homes have sometimes been criticized for offering varying levels of quality in the care they offer because licensed professionals do not typically run them. You need to do some research when selecting a treatment setting.

Psychotherapy. Psychotherapy is a large part of an effective dual diagnosis treatment plan. Cognitive behavioral therapy helps people with dual diagnosis learn how to cope and change ineffective patterns of thinking and behavior, which may influence their risk of substance use.

Medications. Medications are useful for treating mental illnesses. Certain medications can also help people experiencing substance use disorders ease withdrawal symptoms during the detoxification process and help promote recovery.

Self-help and support groups. Dealing with a dual diagnosis can feel challenging and isolating. Support groups allow members to share frustrations, celebrate successes, find referrals for specialists, identify community resources, and swap recovery tips.

PART TWO

What Can I Do to Help Myself?

CHAPTER 9

Understanding the Basics of Mental Health

Our brain needs continuous care to function well. That includes doing certain essential things every day to maintain our emotional health and stability—these are called the *basics of mental health*. These essentials include observing a regular pattern of sleep, diet, and exercise, as well as taking medications as advised, having a daily routine and structure, and maintaining frequent contact with nontoxic friends and family. The basics are outlined in table 9.1. Following them has been shown to have a positive impact on your overall emotional health and mental illness.

Having mental health symptoms may often interfere with your ability to follow these basics. For example, with depression it becomes more difficult to find the energy to exercise, shop for healthy groceries, cook and eat well, or pick up the phone and interact with friends. I urge you to keep at it anyway.

SLEEP

Sleep is essential to restore and repair the effects of the day. Sound sleep optimizes brain function and has a positive effect on your mood disorder and physical health.

Sleep problems (insomnia) often occur during an episode of major depression, anxiety, PTSD, stress, grief, and in the wake of a disaster or pandemic. You may sleep too much, too little, or have interrupted sleep, with frequent awakenings during the night. You may have trouble falling asleep, or you may wake up too early. The quality of your sleep may be affected so that you don't feel rested or restored the next day. Without enough sleep you may become irritable and have difficulty concentrating and doing small tasks.

Changes in your sleep may or may not be fully under your control. They may be related to a physical condition such as sleep apnea or extreme stress. Sleep difficulties may be warning signs or symptoms of your worsening mental illness, which you and your provider can recognize and address. Sleep disruption may also be related to environmental conditions, such as noise level, excess light, or extremes in room temperature. The good news is that you can control some things to help yourself achieve a good night's sleep. Recommended treatment for long-standing insomnia includes two main approaches: cognitive behavioral therapy and sedating medication.

Cognitive behavioral therapy for insomnia (CBT-I), a type of talk therapy, is considered the first-line treatment for sleep problems. It addresses the unhelpful thoughts, beliefs, and behaviors about sleep that contribute to a persistent sleep problem. CBT-I includes restricting the hours you sleep, cognitive therapy to restore and maintain reasonable expectations about sleep, relaxation therapy, and sleep hygiene.

Sleep hygiene is a strategy that helps you reduce behaviors that interfere with sleep or that may increase your excitability or stimulation around bedtime (table 9.2). It's one way to optimize your sleep. Sleep hygiene refers to the personal habits and environmental conditions (what it's like in your bedroom) that affect a person's sleep, including not eating, reading, working, or watching TV in bed and reserving the bed for sleep or sex only. Try to avoid being stimulated at bedtime (by invigorating music, TV, conversations or phone calls, or blue light from electronic devices).

TABLE 9.1 Basics of Mental Health

- Treat any physical illness.

- Get enough sleep:
  - Aim for seven to eight hours of sleep each night.
  - Go to bed and wake up at the same time every day of the week, including nonwork and nonschool days. Keep a regular sleep routine.
  - Keep your sleep environment quiet and relaxing.
  - Reserve the bed for sleep and sex only and no other activities, such as eating, working, reading, watching television, and so on.
  - Track your sleep routine with a sleep diary and share it with your doctor.
  - Follow the sleep hygiene guidelines to promote restful sleep (table 9.2).

- Ensure a healthy diet and nutrition:
  - Eat three healthy, balanced meals each day.
  - Avoid street drugs and alcohol.
  - Limit caffeine intake.
  - For basic nutritional guidelines, see www.choosemyplate.gov and USDA *Dietary Guidelines for Americans, 2020–2025* (table 9.3).

- Use medications as needed:
  - Take all medications as prescribed.
  - Talk to your doctor about the use of vitamins and herbal supplements.

- Exercise regularly:
  - Seek a balance of cardiovascular, strength training, stretching, and relaxation activities three to five days per week.
  - Strive for 150 to 300 minutes of moderate exercise per week or 75 minutes of vigorous exercise per week (see *Physical Activity Guidelines for Americans*, US HHS 2018).

- Maintain regular and positive social contact with your friends and family. Avoid isolation.

- Have a routine and structure to each day:
  - Structure your time each day (but it doesn't have to be rigid).
  - Write your daily tasks and appointments in an electronic or paper agenda.
  - Break large tasks into small steps.
  - Include positive, pleasurable experiences in your day as well as home, family, school, and work responsibilities.

TABLE 9.2 Sleep Hygiene

Recommendations to improve your sleep include the following:

- Keep the same bedtime and wake-up time every day, including on weekends. Set an alarm clock if necessary. Get up and out of bed at the same time every morning, even if you've had a bad night's sleep.
- Avoid napping during the day.
- Develop a relaxing ritual before bedtime. Create downtime during the last 2 hours before sleep and avoid overstimulation.
- Try going to bed only when you are sleepy.
- Avoid watching the clock or lying in bed frustrated at being unable to fall asleep. Turn the clock away from you.
- If you're unable to fall asleep after 20 to 30 minutes, get out of bed. Relax and distract your mind with a quiet activity in another room (music, reading). Return to bed when you feel sleepy.
- Relaxation exercises before bedtime may help. Examples include progressive muscle relaxation, deep breathing, guided imagery, yoga, or meditation.
- Designate a specific "worry time" earlier in the day or evening to sort out any problems. Writing down reminders for the next day helps to clear your mind before bed.
- Use your bed and bedroom only for sleep, sex, or occasional illness. Eliminate nonsleep activities in bed. Use another room for reading, television, work, and eating.
- Limit the use of caffeine during the day and avoid its use after 12:00 p.m. Note that coffee, tea, colas, chocolate, and some medications contain caffeine.
- Avoid or limit the use of nicotine (tobacco) and alcohol during the day. Don't use them within 4 to 6 hours of bedtime.
- Avoid large meals before bedtime, but don't go to bed hungry. If needed, have a light snack.
- Exercise regularly. Avoid strenuous exercise within 4 to 6 hours of bedtime.
- Create a bedroom environment that favors sound sleep. A comfortable bed in a dark, quiet room is recommended. Minimize light, noise, and hot or cold extremes in room temperature. Room-darkening shades, curtains, earplugs, or a sound machine may be helpful.
- Speak with your doctor if you are having continued difficulty with sleep, including falling asleep, staying asleep, and early or frequent awakenings.

Source: Susan J. Noonan, *Managing Your Depression: What You Can Do to Feel Better* (Baltimore, MD: Johns Hopkins University Press, 2013), 8–9. Additional references: American Academy of Sleep Medicine, "Healthy Sleep Habits," updated August 2020, http:// sleepeducation.org/essentials-in-sleep/healthy-sleep-habits; Sleep Foundation, "Sleep Hygiene," updated August 14, 2020, https://www.sleepfoundation.org/sleep-hygiene.

What is enough sleep for me? The amount of sleep required by a person depends in part on age. It varies from infancy, through childhood, to older age. The average amount of sleep required by healthy adults is 7 to 8 hours per night. "Enough sleep" is the amount that makes you feel physically and mentally rested, sharp, not irritable, and able to concentrate, focus, and correctly do small motor tasks.

DIET AND NUTRITION

Feed your body; feed your brain. Eat real food. Food is the fuel that keeps our bodies and brains operating properly and helps to stabilize our emotions. Eating well-balanced healthy meals is one way of taking care of yourself that you have control over. It can make a positive difference in your mental health. When you stray from a healthy regular diet, skip meals, or overeat in response to emotional cues, you become vulnerable to mood changes. You may become irritable and fatigued, and your brain may not function very well.

One trick I use is to have three different colored foods on my plate at each meal (protein, vegetables, etc.).

Eating for energy and balanced mental health means that you have three small to medium meals per day plus one or two healthy snacks as you choose. Don't skip meals. A balanced whole food diet high in nutrient-dense foods including whole fruits, a variety of colorful vegetables, whole grains, beans, fish, poultry, and a small amount of olive oil improves mood and is associated with a lower rate of depression. The Mediterranean Diet is often recommended as a healthy option that is easy to follow and is linked with decreased rates of depression compared to a Western diet.

Dietary Guidelines for Americans, 2020–2025

The USDA *Dietary Guidelines for Americans, 2020–2025* (table 9.3) describe a healthy diet and lifestyle as one that

- emphasizes more whole or minimally processed foods and plant-based foods in a healthy eating pattern across every stage of life (infancy through older adulthood);
- is focused on variety, nutrient density, and the amount of food;
- emphasizes fruits, vegetables, whole grains, and lean protein (lean meats, poultry, fish, beans, eggs, and nuts);
- emphasizes fat-free or low-fat milk and dairy products;
- is low in saturated fats, trans fats, cholesterol, salt (sodium), added sugars, and alcohol;
- meets the *Physical Activity Guidelines for Americans* (available online at US HHS, https://health.gov/our-work /nutrition-physical-activity/physical-activity-guidelines /current-guidelines).

The dietary guidelines display healthy food as portions divided on a dinner plate, with fruits, vegetables, whole grains, lean protein (such as chicken or fish), and a small amount of dairy. Pay attention to portion sizes at home and when you eat out, because they have slowly increased in size over the years at restaurants and in the home. There is an easy-to-use interactive website to help you understand the food portions at USDA, "My Plate," www.choosemyplate.gov. Visit this website for many helpful tips on healthy eating, including menu choices and specific caloric goals for your age and gender. Optimal daily caloric intake depends on your gender, age, current weight, activity level, and goals for maintaining, losing, or gaining weight. This is individual for each person; your family doctor or a dietitian can help you identify your caloric goal.

Sometimes it feels much easier to skip meals or eat fast food, takeout, and prepared foods that are higher in fats and salt and

TABLE 9.3 USDA 2020–2025 Dietary Guidelines for Americans

This list summarizes the key points in maintaining a healthy body and weight.

1. Follow a healthy dietary pattern at every life stage (infancy to older adulthood).
2. Customize nutrient-dense food and beverage choices to reflect personal preference, cultural traditions, and budgetary considerations.
3. Meet food group needs with nutrient-dense foods and beverages and stay within calorie limits. Increase whole grains, vegetables, and whole fruits in your diet.
4. Limit foods and beverages higher in added sugars, saturated fat, and sodium, and limit alcoholic beverages.

The core elements that make up a healthy dietary pattern include the following:

1. Vegetables of all types–dark green; red and orange; beans, peas, and lentils; starchy; and other vegetables
2. Fruits, especially whole fruit
3. Grains, at least half of which are whole grain (barley, oats, brown rice, quinoa) instead of refined grains (white flour and white rice)
4. Dairy, including fat-free or low-fat milk, yogurt, and cheese, or lactose-free versions and fortified soy beverages and yogurt as alternatives
5. Protein foods, including lean meats, poultry, and eggs; seafood; beans, peas, and lentils; and nuts, seeds, and soy products
6. Oils, including vegetable oils and oils in food, such as seafood, avocado, nuts, in moderation

Healthy eating habits include the following:

1. Focus on the total number of calories consumed. Monitor your food intake.
2. Be aware of portion size: choose smaller portions or lower-calorie options.
3. Eat less than 10 percent of your calories per day from added sugars (12.5 teaspoons per day).
4. Limit daily sodium (salt) intake to less than 2,300 milligrams per day.
5. Eat less than 10 percent of calories from saturated fats (butter, cream, cheese, fatty meats) by replacing them with monounsaturated and poly-unsaturated fatty acids (olive oil, canola oil, walnuts, flax seeds, sunflower seeds, fish such as salmon, trout, or mackerel).
6. Choose fat-free or low-fat milk and milk products (milk, yogurt, cheese) or soy.
7. Use alcohol in moderation. The limit should be 0–2 alcoholic drinks per day for adult men and 0–1 alcoholic drink per day for adult women.
8. Eliminate foods that contain synthetic sources of trans fats, such as partially hydrogenated oils (read food labels).
9. Stay physically active and meet the *Physical Activity Guidelines for Americans* (US HHS 2018).

Source: US Department of Agriculture and US Department of Health and Human Services, *Dietary Guidelines for Americans, 2020–2025*, 9th ed. (Washington, DC: Government Printing Office, 2020), https://www.dietaryguidelines.gov/sites/default/files/2020-12/Dietary _Guidelines_for_Americans_2020-2025.pdf.

not as healthy for you or your brain. Grocery shopping and cooking may seem overwhelming, but try to remind yourself how important it is for your mental and physical health. You need the nutrients from a healthy diet as fuel for your body and brain to operate at their best. You may find it easier to stick to a healthy diet when you plan ahead. Choose which nutritious foods you like and balance your preferences.

PHYSICAL EXERCISE

Move more, sit less. Exercise is medicine. Physical exercise is good for your brain, body, and soul. And it's something we all have control over. Moderate to vigorous physical activity improves mood, enriches the quality of sleep, and promotes improvements in mild to moderate depressive and anxiety symptoms.

The benefits of physical exercise as a treatment for mental illness are that it

- increases a brain chemical called BDNF that promotes the growth of new brain cells
- helps to regulate brain chemicals (neurotransmitters)
- helps to keep the level of stress hormones normal, relieving stress
- increases feelings of confidence, self-esteem, competence, and sense of mastery
- has a positive effect on your mood
- improves your sense of well-being
- releases the "feel good" hormones (endorphins)
- improves the quality of your sleep, which in turn improves your mood disorder
- helps to overcome the inertia and sedentary lifestyle that often comes with depression
- increases your social contacts (in an exercise class or in neighborhood or health club interactions)

- builds endurance and physical strength, which combats fatigue
- helps manage your weight

It may be more difficult to follow a regular exercise routine during social isolation or a pandemic. You have to be committed to doing it and look for creative ways to move. Walk the dog, play in the yard with your kids, or quickly walk up and down the stairs in your home ten times in a row. Do a fitness walk outdoors with a friend or neighbor, wearing a face mask or keeping a social distance of 6 feet apart. Maybe you can get multicolored resistance bands or a set of handheld weights online to keep up with strength training at home. If you're working from home, sitting at your computer as I am now, try to get up periodically and move around. Or participate in a phone call or Zoom meeting while standing—nobody will really know or mind. That small interruption will improve your productivity as well.

What counts as physical exercise? Basically, any intentional, repetitive, organized movement of the body that uses energy and raises your heart rate and breathing is exercise—that is, when you get sweaty and out of breath.

The American College of Sports Medicine considers a regular physical exercise program essential for most adults. It's recommended that we do

- *aerobic activities* that increase our heart rate and breathing;
- *strength activities*, which means moving in a controlled way against a force or resistance that builds and maintains bones and muscle; and
- *balance and stretching activities* that increase physical stability and flexibility, such as yoga, tai chi, or basic stretches.

The physical activity guidelines recommend that adults get

- at least 150 to 300 minutes of moderate intensity physical activity per week (30 minutes of moderate activity

5 times a week) and muscle strength training on two or
more days of the week *or*

- at least 75 minutes of vigorous intensity physical activity
  per week (25 minutes of vigorous activity 3 times a week)
  and strength training on two or more days of the week
  and
- flexibility and balance exercises at least twice per week.

To balance out our physical activities, stretch and flexibility,
balance, relaxation, and perhaps a meditation routine have also
been found to be helpful.

The guidelines have separate activity sections with specifi-
cations for children, older adults over age 65, physical activity
during pregnancy and postpartum, and for adults who have a
chronic health condition.

Depression and anxiety symptoms may make it more difficult to start and stick with an exercise program. These symptoms include loss of interest in activities, decreased physical
and mental energy, decreased motivation, and loss of focus and
concentration. It's hard to make healthy choices when you don't
feel well. Some people believe that they don't have enough time
for physical exercise, that they're too tired or embarrassed, that
it's boring or won't help, or that other things in life are more
important. I urge you to keep at it.

How to Get Started

Choose an exercise activity that you enjoy, or used to enjoy, that
is realistic and that you can do regularly. Some ideas are found in
table 9.4. Once you pick your exercise program, sticking with it is
the most important part. *How do you do that when you're isolated
or depressed?* That's a challenge. Make exercise part of your daily
routine and schedule it as a key part of your day. Here is where
action precedes motivation. This means that you should start your
exercise program now and keep at it, even if you don't really feel
like doing it. The motivation for doing it will come later.

TABLE 9.4 Get Started with Exercise and Keep It Going

- Do what you enjoy or used to enjoy. Do something that is fun.
- Assess what type of exercise resources are available to you. Look for a safe area to walk in your neighborhood. When the COVID-19 pandemic has passed, find out if there is a community center or health club facility available to you with exercise classes or equipment. For now, consider whether you have or can invest in home exercise equipment. See what kind of social supports are available to keep you motivated to exercise.
- Plan a specific and realistic activity that you can do. Define the type of activity, how often you will do it, and for how long (frequency and duration).
- Make exercise a priority in your day and a key part of your daily routine.
- Believe that the exercise will benefit you—this will make it easier to do.
- List the pros and cons of exercising compared to having a sedentary lifestyle.
- Come up with your own personal reasons for exercising.
- Exercise with a partner (a walking partner or people in a class) while wearing a mask and maintaining social distancing guidelines— you will have to be accountable to them to show up and exercise together. This is a good social support.
- Consider having a personal trainer help you set up a program, then monitor and motivate you. This can be done virtually.
- Identify and address any barriers ahead of time, such as the time of day, your energy level, balancing other obligations, being too busy, too tired, too sick, bored, embarrassed, and so forth.
- Work toward a goal that has personal meaning. This could be a walking or running distance or length of time, or a specific exercise accomplishment.
- Train for a charity event (such as a walk-, run-, or bike-a-thon).
- Track your progress in a journal or log and review it periodically.
- Focus on the activity and not on your performance. Try not to make comparisons to your past or others' performance.
- As you get stronger, vary your activity so that you avoid boredom and repetitive injury.
- Give yourself credit for what you can do now.

If you have not exercised in a while, start slowly and gradually build up your time and effort. Commit to walking briskly around the block for 10 minutes each day, and then gradually increase the amount of time you walk each week. Set realistic, achievable goals. Incorporate small changes into your daily activities, such as walking more places, taking the stairs instead of the elevator, or getting off the subway or bus two stops earlier.

As you keep up your exercise program, your strength, endurance, and energy level will improve. The more you do, the stronger you will become, and the more likely you will continue the activity. The best advice I have read is to get fit and continue to challenge yourself, raising the bar periodically. The more fit you are physically, the more resilient your brain will become, and the better it will function.

AVOID ISOLATION

Social isolation and living through the COVID-19 pandemic may cause you to experience depression, anxiety, grief, or PTSD, and with that there is a tendency to withdraw further from the activities of your daily life and avoid contact with friends and family. Some people tend to isolate themselves and prefer to stay at home, not get dressed, or answer the telephone—it's easier that way. I urge you to avoid the temptation to cut yourself off from others, even during the COVID-19 pandemic. Social isolation and lack of social support increase the risk of developing depression and may prolong episodes of depression. Keeping up with social contacts may help maintain your emotional well-being and protect against depression and other mental health problems. Interacting with others provides many benefits, such as a feeling of acceptance, increased self-esteem, a chance for friendship and fun, and access to someone who can provide support if you need it.

> *Dr. Douglas Katz and I spoke about the value of having people in our lives. He points out that those who live alone during the pandemic seem to be faring worse than people who have supports in the home. When people have others around them, they can create some kind of simulation or version of the life they once had. They can engage in structure and daily routines that resemble their former lives. But for people who live alone, there's just a vast expanse of time and little to do with that time. That leaves a lot of time for rumination (thinking repeatedly of and dwelling on negative, unpleasant experiences), thinking about past regrets, what will happen once the pandemic ends, and other unproductive thoughts.*
>
> Author interview with Dr. Douglas Katz, December 28, 2020

People have found many creative and safe ways to get needed human contact using social media and social distancing. For example, during the early months of the pandemic, I had a FaceTime Sunday brunch with a friend, where we set up our electronic devices in our kitchens and chatted and visited as we each cooked our respective meals and ate together. Others have had game nights with friends over Zoom and book clubs and holiday parties on social media. I even

Action precedes motivation. This is the mantra that keeps me going.

attended a beautiful wedding virtually where I was able to see everything in much greater detail than if I had been physically present. Once the pandemic restrictions have lifted, remember that there is no substitute for in-person human contact.

Avoiding isolation when depressed or anxious can be a challenge. The first step is to recognize when it is happening. Do not wait until you feel like it to get out and be with others. Push yourself a little and just do it, a bit at a time. Make a point of returning telephone calls from friends and family who are helpful and positive. Don't substitute text messaging for real-time phone calls and in-person contact with others, although in this time of COVID, I urge you to take caution. Throughout 2020, restrictions have been in place to interact only with those in your immediate household, but this will not be forever.

Set your expectations to do the activities you can do now and modify them as needed. Get out of the house. Do one or two errands at a time, not a dozen. Say hello to the store clerk. For now, walk for 10 minutes around the block rather than tackling your usual exercise routine. Eventually, it will all become easier to do.

A written routine and schedule can help you manage the tendency to withdraw. You can do this on paper or on an electronic device. That way, you have something concrete to follow for the times when you are tempted to isolate. The key is to stick to your schedule even when you don't feel like it. Hold yourself accountable for following through. Then give yourself credit for this accomplishment.

ROUTINE AND STRUCTURE

Routine and consistency in daily life help make your life more manageable and in control. It is thought that small changes in one's daily routine place stress on the body's ability to maintain stability, and that those with mood disorders have a more difficult time adapting to these changes in routine. Paying close attention to daily routines, and to the positive and negative events that influence those routines and cause you stress, increases your stability.

Schedule your time each day and try to follow that schedule, but also be flexible with yourself. Keep track of your responsibilities and activities in a calendar or agenda book—electronic or paper, whatever you prefer, just as long as you will use it. Plan your time each day to include a balance of these things:

- Responsibilities and obligations: things you do at work, home, school, with family
- Daily self-care:
  - meals and nutrition
  - medications, treatments, therapy
  - personal care: showering, shaving, brushing your teeth, getting dressed
  - sleep
  - exercise
- Social contacts—being with people you like has a positive effect on your mood, so keep in regular contact with people and situations in a COVID-safe way
- Positive experiences:
  - pleasant and pleasurable activities: it is not enough to eliminate the negative experiences in life—you also need to include positive and pleasurable experiences
  - mastery of activities: activities that are somewhat difficult for you to do and are a challenge give a sense of being competent and effective—learning a new skill or overcoming an obstacle is one way to achieve mastery
  - purpose in life: include activities that give you a sense of purpose in your daily schedule

As you plan your day, try to keep your tasks and activities
- Prioritized: understand what is most important for you to do.
- Measurable: put a time frame around each activity (instead of open-ended time).
- Attainable and realistic: start with the things that you can do now, in your current state:
  - pace yourself
  - break large complex tasks down into small steps that are more realistic and manageable

- don't overschedule—this creates more stress and the
  potential for failure
- learn to set limits and say no when you are over-
  extended
• Concrete and specific: clearly define each goal and task.
• Flexible: understand where you are and what you can do
  at any given time and modify your schedule as needed.
  Do not compare your current self and abilities to past
  levels of performance or functioning.

Finding Effective Professional Mental Health Care

Although you are doing the best you can, at some point you may find that you need the assistance of a mental health professional to help you through a difficult time. Any persistent change in your usual self that causes distress, significantly interferes with your daily functioning, and lasts for two weeks or longer signals that professional mental health treatment would be helpful.

When considering professional treatment for any mental health condition, keep in mind that there is no quick fix or magic pill to whisk away your distress and emotional pain. It most likely took a long time for you to get to this place and will take a while to understand and unravel it. Treatment requires a lot of hard work and can feel frustrating at times. Therapy sessions can open painful wounds that can create dread and anxiety and be too raw and difficult sometimes, with discomfort that might last for days or weeks afterward. Medications take weeks before any signs of improvement are obvious, which requires extraordinary patience. Your task is to be as patient as possible and try to recognize small moments of progress.

The mental health impact of social isolation and a pandemic such as COVID-19 has increased the number of persons in need of mental health treatment. It highlights the current inequities in care affecting most health care systems and the challenges in obtaining access to professional mental health care. One solution proposed is the *collaborative care model* of treatment. This is an integrated and coordinated method of delivering mental health care involving multidisciplinary clinical care teams made up of a social worker or nurse who manages the overall care, a primary care physician (PCP) who provides care based on the recommendations of a mental health professional, a psychiatrist as the consultant, and sometimes other specialists. The collaborative care model has been studied and proven effective in the treatment of depression, anxiety, PTSD, and other mental health conditions.

This model of health care delivery can also operate effectively using telemedicine for patient visits and virtual conferences between providers. Telemedicine is an online virtual appoint-

> Since the COVID-19 pandemic began, Dr. Sheila Rauch has observed changes in how people are dealing with it: changes over time and changes within a person. She has seen people who had prior mental health issues respond in different ways. Some of them are able to reach out and get the resources they need through telehealth or telemedicine (virtual appointments) or through other systems of care through community or family. Some are more isolated (and unable to seek mental health care)—they have had real increases in their risk of mental illness and in the severity of their PTSD, depression, or substance use. Dr. Rauch sees isolation as the biggest issue affecting mental health.
>
> She believes that people who have had mental health diagnoses for a shorter amount of time, such as those experiencing their first mental health symptoms, are probably going to respond to treatments more quickly, with less impairment than what comes from experiencing a mental health disorder for the long term without treatment. That results in less impact on their family, their income, and overall financial situation, but it doesn't make it any less serious. She sees a lot of strength in her patients even though many of them are struggling.
>
> ———
> Author interview with Dr. Sheila Rauch, December 21, 2020

ment where both patient and provider communicate over a computer. (See "Virtual Visits" below for more on telemedicine.) In this current pandemic era, with increased demand for mental health services, it enables a psychiatrist to treat and consult on a larger number of affected people. Collaborative care delivered virtually also lends itself well to those in rural or underserved areas, as it eliminates any geographic barriers to receiving care. And collaboration with a PCP ensures that the whole person's needs will be addressed, including any physical medical problems associated with their mental illness.

Caring for those persons who have complex emotional and physical medical problems is another challenge. Many experts endorse assembling an unofficial virtual "team" of outpatient providers from different specialties all working together and communicating with each other in caring for the person in distress. This is often done remotely by telephone or electronic communication—the team does not actually meet together. The care team might include a psychiatrist, psychologist, primary care physician, and other specialists as needed (oncologist or other cancer doctors, etc.). Dr. Michael Sharpe of Oxford University has called this team "the pit crew," using an analogy from the car racing world.

MAKING THE DIAGNOSIS OF MENTAL ILLNESS

There are no blood tests for stress, depression, or anxiety, and no brain scans are readily available outside a research setting. An illness of the brain leads to changes in the chemicals, cells, and structure of the brain that until recently have been difficult to observe, test for, and measure. This difficulty has meant that people have a hard time believing the disorders are real, adding to the stigma of mental illness.

In clinical practice, to make the diagnosis of a mental health condition, your doctor will take your vital signs (heart rate, blood pressure), do a basic physical exam, and ask you a detailed series of questions about how you are feeling and what kind of symptoms you are having. Sometimes, with your permission, information from family members and loved ones is also obtained. Topics asked about include your sleep, appetite, weight, interests, daily activities, work or school, social supports, and thoughts of harming yourself. Your health care provider might ask if you are able to function in your daily activities and responsibilities; how much sleep you are getting; whether you are eating three healthy meals a day; whom you interact with regularly; whether you are still involved with previously enjoyed hobbies or sports and exercise; and whether you have ever thought about harming yourself or not wanting to be here—things like that.

Your physician will then test your ability to think, reason, express yourself, and remember things by asking a series of simple questions that demonstrate these skills, while paying attention to your mood, behavior, and general appearance. For example, your PCP might ask you to explain a simple phrase or remember five specific objects five minutes later. All of this is called a *mental health assessment*, which is the next step in diagnosing a mental illness. You will also be asked about your family's medical history to determine whether you have any relatives with a mental illness or a contributing medical problem. Next, blood and urine tests will be done to make sure that no other physical problem is causing your illness, such as a thyroid condition or street drugs in your system (these would appear on a toxicology screen).

TYPES OF MENTAL HEALTH PROVIDERS

When you're ready to seek professional mental health care, you can start with your PCP or family doctor, who will ask you questions about how you're feeling and doing. They will assess your situation; evaluate your emotional distress, anxiety, grief, or depression briefly; and either begin treatment right away or refer you to a colleague who specializes in treating people who have mental health problems. It may take a while to make an accurate diagnosis and to find a mental health provider with whom you feel comfortable. Some PCPs are experienced in treating early depression, anxiety, and grief, and that may be just what you need. But more severe types of these mental illnesses may require a mental health specialist.

Choosing a mental health provider depends on your needs. There are several different types of providers, each with different training and skills. Selecting the category of professional is the first step. The next decision depends in part on who is practicing in your local area; their availability; and to a certain extent, your insurance coverage (for example, which providers are in your insurance plan's network and are therefore more affordable).

The different types of mental health professionals who are qualified to treat emotional distress, depression, anxiety, grief, and PTSD often work together as a team. The most common providers are listed here, although others might contribute to your care:

- *Psychiatrists*: medical doctors (MDs or DOs) who are specialty trained, licensed, and board certified to treat mental illnesses such as major depression, bipolar disorder, anxiety, and other conditions. They are the mental health providers who evaluate you and prescribe medications such as antidepressants.
- *Clinical psychologists*: master's (MS) or doctoral degree (PhD or PsyD) specialists trained and licensed in evaluating and treating mental illnesses using various kinds of talk therapy, or psychotherapy. Psychologists are sometimes referred to as therapists. Different types of psychotherapy exist, and each has a different focus and purpose.

A psychologist will know which type is suitable for you. Talk therapy can help you cope with this illness, understand yourself better, learn healthy ways to manage stress, make sound life decisions, and adjust to major losses and life transitions. Talk therapy can be done in a one-to-one setting or in small groups of people with similar problems.

- *Licensed clinical social workers* (LICSWs or LCSWs): they also provide talk therapy to individuals or in groups. They cannot prescribe medications.
- *Nurse practitioners* (NPs): nurses with advanced training who can specialize in psychiatric disorders and are licensed to prescribe antidepressants and other psychiatric medications.

THE RELATIONSHIP WITH YOUR MENTAL HEALTH PROVIDER

The success of your treatment, particularly psychotherapy or talk therapy, depends on building a trusting relationship with a therapist or psychiatrist who is a good fit for you. How do you find this person? That answer varies among individuals. One place to start is to ask your primary care doctor for a recommendation. Depending on who is available in your geographic area, you may be referred to a clinical psychologist, licensed therapist, licensed clinical social worker, and/or a psychiatrist. Try to find one who specializes in treating patients who have symptoms similar to yours, such as depression, anxiety, or PTSD. If you live near a large teaching hospital, most academic psychiatry departments have specialized and separated divisions for depression, anxiety, and PTSD, and they can refer you to a staff member. Get several names and then interview each one face to face to see if you feel comfortable speaking with this person—this may take several visits. Not everyone will be a good match for you, so keep looking until you find someone you think you can open up to. It's okay and expected to do this.

Don't be afraid to ask questions of the people you interview: Inquire about their professional training and background. Make sure that the person you choose will coordinate your care with your other doctors (psychiatrist, therapist, family doctor, etc.). Find out if they can schedule your appointments around your work hours. Ask about the method of payment and whether your health insurance company will pay for it. Ask if they have particular experience with your cultural background and primary language. If you live in a remote area, check out whether the provider can communicate with you by telephone or through a virtual session or other online options.

WHAT MAKES A GOOD MENTAL HEALTH PROVIDER?

There are many different kinds of therapists and psychiatrists, each with a particular style, personality, training, and area of interest. They may practice different types of psychotherapy (talk therapy) or psychiatry. Those differences do not prevent them from delivering good quality care.

You should expect that a good therapist or psychiatrist
- listens and pays attention
- is empathetic and understanding
- is not judgmental or dismissive
- shows respect
- builds trust over time
- offers sound professional advice
- maintains boundaries
- offers treatment recommendations customized for your individual clinical needs and person
- does not impose their personal biases or viewpoints on you

- helps you to see your way through a problem and does
  not do it for you
- builds on your strengths
- offers you a regular appointment, ideally at the same
  time and day
- begins and ends appointments on time
- does not take telephone calls or allow other distractions
  during your appointment
- is available to you by text or telephone after hours for
  emergencies
- maintains your privacy and confidentiality

WHAT MAKES A GOOD PATIENT?

What do you need to do to get the most benefit from your psychotherapy and psychiatric treatment? Show by your actions
that you are interested in and committed to the treatment. Participating in therapy is a two-way street, and you have to do a
lot of the hard work. You also need to keep up a good professional relationship with your provider. Helping yourself in this
way provides the best chance of recovery and of staying well.

These guidelines will help you be successful:

- Follow all treatments as prescribed. This includes taking
  medications and acting on other recommended therapies.
- Keep your appointments as scheduled. Do not skip
  appointments or cancel them at the last minute unless
  there is an emergency.
- Go to your appointments on time and stay for the entire
  session.
- Arrive sober. Do not show up to your appointment under
  the influence of alcohol or drugs.
- Be honest with your therapist and psychiatrist.
- Make an effort.

- Do the "homework" assignments that your therapist asks you to do.
- Come prepared for each session with an idea of what you would like to discuss or work on with your provider.
- Turn off your cellphone, tablet, and other electronic devices during your appointment.
- Listen.
- Pay attention to the conversation. Catch yourself if you begin to daydream off the subject.
- Take notes if you are having trouble concentrating or remembering what is being discussed.
- Show respect.
- Maintain boundaries. This is a professional relationship, not a casual friendship.
- Control your anger and outbursts during the session. If anger is a problem for you, your therapist will make addressing it part of your treatment plan.
- Learn to trust your clinician and understand that they have your best interest in mind.
- Avoid making phone calls to your therapist unless the situation is urgent.
- Call your mental health provider or go to the nearest Emergency Department if you are feeling unsafe or suicidal.

SHARED DECISION MAKING

When working with your health care and mental health care providers, I encourage you to participate in *shared decision making*. Shared decision making is a process in which you and your clinician work together to make decisions regarding your care. You as patient are invited, in fact expected, to ask questions, and your opinion, values, and preferences for treatment are acknowledged and respected. Together you and your provider select diagnostic tests, treatments, and care plans based on clinical evidence while

Shared decision making is the model of patient-centered care.

balancing the risks and benefits with your individual (and informed) preferences and values. Shared decision making educates and empowers you to make a choice that best suits you. It gives you a sense of control. The more you understand your treatment options, the better the chance you will be able to follow through on the recommendations that are consistent with your preferences, leading to greater overall success.

CULTURAL DIFFERENCES IN MENTAL HEALTH CARE

Culture refers to the learned values, beliefs, principles, traditions, social norms, guidelines or rules of behavior, and way of life that are shared among members of a particular group of people. Culture directs how one thinks about, views, and interacts with the world. For example, it defines certain observed religious practices, dietary patterns, music preferences, social roles, and customs, such as the traditional wearing of a kilt in Scotland, a cowboy hat in the western United States, or a kimono in Japan. Many cultures exist, centered on a wide variety of things, such as ancestry, race, and ethnicity; gender; religious beliefs; educational affiliation; military experience; common interests; team sports; and others.

Cultural differences affect the experience of social isolation and loneliness. Some cultures have a strong family and community connection that can offset the impact of isolation, including during an infectious disease pandemic. Imposed isolation, however, may be felt more strongly in an individual raised in this kind of environment. Other cultures are not as connected, and the experience of isolation and loneliness can become a chronic problem.

Culture molds how people regard their health, illness, and hardships; frames the meaning that people give to that illness; directs their coping styles; and determines how a person feels about relying on others. Culture influences one's beliefs about health promotion practices; the causes of disease; how illness and pain are experienced, expressed, and talked about; whether and where a person seeks help; what type of help or treatment they prefer and seek; and what kind of support they have around them. Belief systems vary among cultures, including beliefs related to health care, such as traditional Chinese medicine and the health conventions of Native peoples and those of India and Afghanistan, for example, where there is little to no distinction between the mind and body, in contrast with Western medicine. It's also related to a person's level of health literacy—how much they know about diseases and treatments—which may vary among cultural groups.

Every culture has its own way of regarding mental health, which affects how we express our thoughts, emotions, and behaviors. Culture determines how people feel about their emotional symptoms and whether one considers their feelings a public or private matter. For example, some cultures regard mental health challenges as a weakness and something to hide, while others are more open and accepting. Shame around mental illness is a powerful force in some cultures, such as in many Asian societies. And for many African American, Asian, and other communities, there is growing stigma around mental health conditions, with fear of others finding out and of being ostracized from community. Mental illness is often regarded as private "family business" and kept hidden so as not to reflect poorly on the person or their family. This can make it harder for those struggling to talk openly and ask for help. Cultural factors also determine how much support someone gets from their family and community for a mental health condition.

(continued)

One example of differences across cultures is in the way people experience and express anxiety and depression. In a culture where these mental health conditions are recognized and not considered taboo, and where psychological concepts and terms are familiar, one might openly describe feelings of anxiety and depression using those specific words. In other cultures, such as in some Asian societies, the language to convey mental health conditions does not exist. In addition, some people may focus more on physical symptoms such as headache or back pain rather than appreciating their anxiety. And, in contrast to white Americans, Latino and Black Americans more commonly connect mental illness with spiritual, moral, and social beliefs, leading them to seek different coping strategies and nonclinicians for counsel, such as clergy and cultural healers.

Sadly yet realistically, traditional mental health approaches may not adequately fit the needs of a culturally diverse community. Access to effective mental health care may be affected by language barriers; health literacy and unfamiliarity with the concept of mental health care; mistrust of health care services and clinicians; health insurance status; immigration status; racism and discrimination; negative personal experiences or past trauma; and strong religious overtones. Mental health care must be tailored to the individual—aligned with their identity, culture, and set of experiences.

When looking for mental health treatment, the universal goal is to find a provider who understands your specific experiences and concerns, as well as the role that cultural differences play in the diagnosis and treatment of a mental health condition, and who incorporates cultural needs and differences into your care. This will promote an effective therapeutic relationship. Care must include cultural awareness (sensitivity to the similarities and differences between two different cultures) and cultural competence (having an awareness, understanding, and acceptance of cultural differences without the clinician using their own beliefs and behaviors as the norm).

TYPES OF PROFESSIONAL MENTAL HEALTH TREATMENT

Various types of mental health treatment have proved effective for people who experience anxiety, depression, grief, or PTSD. It can be delivered in an office or clinic setting (outpatient) or in the psychiatric unit of a hospital (inpatient). Sadly, in 2019, prior to the pandemic, it was found that in the United States, more than half of those who experienced mild or moderate mental illness did not receive any professional mental health treatment (psychiatrist or clinical psychologist; SAMHSA 2020).

The most effective type of treatment depends on your symptoms, medical history, and, to some extent, the type of therapy (if any) you've had in the past. It can be difficult to predict how any one person will respond to which treatment. You may have to try several medications or types of treatment before finding the most effective one for your needs with minimal side effects.

Medication therapy and psychotherapy alone are each effective in treating depression and anxiety and in reducing the risk of relapse and recurrence. Sometimes medication alone is sufficient, sometimes talk therapy alone is sufficient, and sometimes a combination is needed. The most effective therapy, in all but the earliest forms of depression, often involves working with both a psychiatrist for medication and a therapist for talk therapy.

Talk Therapy

Talk therapy, or psychotherapy, is a type of guided therapeutic conversation that focuses on a person's psychological and emotional problems, distorted thinking, and troublesome behaviors. It can help you cope with your illness, understand yourself better, learn healthy ways to manage stress, make sound life decisions, and adjust to major life losses and transitions. Psychotherapy offers a broader range of benefits than medications do, such as improving your level of functioning, diminishing residual symptoms, targeting specific symptoms (such as guilt, hopelessness, and pessimism), teaching coping skills, improving interpersonal relationships, and targeting different brain sites. The effects of psychotherapy are long lasting and sustained beyond the end of treatment. Talk therapy can be done one to one or in a group setting. See chapter 11 for a detailed discussion of talk therapy.

Virtual Visits

Social isolation and the COVID-19 pandemic have made in-person access to mental health professionals challenging. Out of concern for social distancing during the pandemic, many health care professionals have looked to alternative ways of connecting. The same may be true for people who live in rural areas where fewer mental health providers are available; they often live a great distance away, and the providers' schedules are often overbooked because of the need to cover large geographic areas.

One recent option that has proved to be remarkably effective is a virtual visit, an online appointment similar to Skype or FaceTime, usually conducted on a computer using an application called Zoom. This is known as *telemedicine* and has been found useful by most clinicians, including mental health professionals (psychiatrists, psychologists, social workers, and others). It's favored by many patients and clients because of the efficiency (no taking time from your day to drive and park) and discretion (friends and colleagues will never know of your mental health appointment). While some feel it lacks a certain level of personal connection, research suggests that virtual talk

Telemedicine is not the same as telehealth, *which is a general term for a broad array of technologies and tactics that deliver virtual medical visits as well as other online health services and health education.*

My conversation with Dr. Sheila Rauch turned to the ongoing nature and stressors of the pandemic as it strains the mental health system. In response to this, she has collaborated on a project to develop a new "phased approach" to COVID-19 mental health treatment for the ADAA (Anxiety and Depression Association of America). It's a guide designed for policy and decision making around trauma, such as this pandemic, and how needs change over time. Dr. Rauch and her colleagues' proposal aids health care systems and programs in their planning efforts to address the mental health treatment needs of health care workers and others related to the COVID-19 pandemic and to prepare and plan for the continued needs of patients, communities, and health care staff.

The phased approach considers patients in three different phases of exposure to trauma (initial phase after exposure, up to three months, and long term) and describes different levels of mental health treatment intervention within each phase (health care system or community, self-care, and professional mental health care level). This initiative is encouraging because it aims to most efficiently get help to people at the level that they need and at the time that they need it.

Author interview with Dr. Sheila Rauch December 21, 2020

therapy (psychotherapy) using telemedicine provides outcomes that are comparable to in-person visits for several mental health conditions. Medicare and private insurers have recently authorized payment of telemedicine for medical and mental health visits. Licensure, HIPAA, and privacy issues, which may have been a concern in the past, have also been addressed.

Prior to the COVID-19 pandemic, licensed clinical psychologists used telemedicine in about 7 percent of their patient encounters; this rose to 85 percent during the pandemic. Telemedicine enables clinicians to meet their patients' mental health needs while adhering to safety restrictions to limit COVID-19 virus transmission. It is not meant to fully replace in-person appointments when the crisis is over; it is estimated that telemedicine usage in mental health will drop to 67 percent when the concerns of the pandemic end.

> *In our interview, Dr. Douglas Katz brought up his thoughts on the merits of virtual therapy and a realization that one positive aspect of the COVID-19 pandemic is our undeniable ability to adapt. Dr. Katz has observed that virtual therapy has opened doors that weren't there before, and that people have taken to it quite well. For example, he now has a better sense of the patient's experience when alone in their own homes and familiar environment, which is different from when they are able to "get it together and show up" in an office setting.*
>
> *When at home, people often have a sense of overwhelming dread, sadness, and anxiety, as well as an incredible desire to escape from their emotional pain that he can now directly observe during a virtual appointment. The escape often involves pushing away the laundry, the showering, doing the dishes, and so forth, and just retreating, sometimes into sleep or the internet. In receiving support and doing therapy virtually from home, some persons may now come to see themselves as capable of doing those things they had avoided. Virtual therapy provides an opportunity for clinician and patient to do things together never before possible and has enabled Dr. Katz to practice at a more enhanced level.*
>
> *Virtual therapy has also made treatment more accessible to many. For example, those who have depression or overwhelming anxiety may be inclined to miss an in-person appointment when their condition is severe and they can't get it together to show up, yet they are frequently able to engage in a virtual session. There are fewer cancellations and missed appointments. This is a huge benefit of Zoom and other technologies during the pandemic and into the future.*

> *Dr. Katz points out that, as a provider, establishing trust and rapport virtually is more difficult with a new patient, although not impossible; it's easier with an established patient. Some subtle quality or nonverbal cues may be missing in the online interaction. It just may take more time and effort. And there are some, such as some elderly, who find the technology daunting, so virtual appointments are not working out for them.*
>
> Author interview with Dr. Douglas Katz, December 28, 2020.

A virtual appointment can be a good and an effective experience for patient and provider, enabling private therapeutic conversations from any location, including home. It has also allowed for some creative encounters not available in a mental health office setting. Seeing you in your usual environment such as your home enables the clinician to obtain valuable insight into your life and try novel therapies not previously conceived of. I personally believe that it works the best when you and your provider have already met and have established a working relationship. Yet it has been thought to work well on first and early mental health appointments.

Reliance on technology using telemedicine and virtual conferencing, however, may be a limitation in those who do not have the technical skills (technical literacy) or a personal computer or WiFi connection necessary to access medical and mental health visits confidentially. In such situations, alternate methods of remote communication can be used, such as a telephone if available. But this does not address the needs of the disenfranchised, the homeless, or those living in shelters and group homes who don't have access to technology. It's an area in need of improvement.

A Collaborative Intervention

Dr. Thea Gallagher has seen a wide range of mental health issues, including depression, anxiety, and more. She's involved in an intervention as part of the wellness program for health care workers at the University of Pennsylvania called Penn COBALT, which aims to break the stigma around receiving mental health treatment and decrease the reluctance to accept intervention. Dr. Gallagher and colleagues have created a spectrum of offerings, including resilience coaching, support groups, individual support, coping tools, podcasts, and so forth, with an example and tone being set by the leadership from the top down. She believes that "it's helpful if people who haven't experienced it are open to talk about their experiences as peer to another, so then it doesn't seem nearly as offensive or frightening."

Dr. Gallagher believes in the value of human connection and small talk, which is lacking during social isolation. Some of the interventions that she has introduced across the health system include "in the beginning of meetings, having a time where people maybe share a funny story or talk about what they did on the weekend. Really kind of trying to introduce that and really being mindful about reaching out to people about things other than work and saying, How are things? and acknowledging people for what they're doing well. We're not used to giving people positive praise, and we need to keep doing that. It makes people feel acknowledged. I think isolation also comes out when we don't feel like we have significance or impact, or that we're not acknowledged."

Author interview with Dr. Thea Gallagher, January 15, 2021

Medications

Many different types of medications can be used to treat depression, anxiety, and other mental health conditions. They work in different ways, and some persons respond better to one category of drug than another, but that's hard to know beforehand and may be different for each person. The choice of medication is based on your particular combination of symptoms and any medical problems you have that may interfere with the drug. If you experience depression, it may realistically take several weeks, or months, to see the effects of medication or other mental health treatment. That can be frustrating and requires setting realistic expectations and a lot of patience on everybody's part. At times, more than one medication is required, or a switch to another category of drug is indicated based on your response and set of symptoms. The greatest challenge for you is the ability to tolerate seemingly unbearable symptoms while waiting for the treatment or medications to work.

Somatic Treatments

Somatic treatments are those that are physically applied to the body and have an effect on the brain; several are described here as treatment for depression. One treatment option sometimes offered when medications do not work well, are not tolerated, or cannot be used for medical reasons is electroconvulsive therapy, or ECT (once called shock therapy). This treatment is usually given for depression in select patients, including the elderly. While under deep but brief sedation, a very low electric current is sent for a few seconds to the brain through electrodes, small sticky pads, which are placed on your scalp. Electrodes transmit the current to the mood center of your brain. Stimulating the brain in this way has been a very effective treatment for many in changing how they feel. ECT is usually given three times a week for several weeks.

It may sound scary, but ECT does not hurt, and you are totally unaware of the process. Some people may have a mild headache for a few hours afterward. Others may lose a portion of their memory from around the time of the treatment. Most people find their depression symptoms improve noticeably after the first few treatments.

Another proven effective treatment in some people who experience depression is repetitive transcranial magnetic stimulation (rTMS). This procedure uses a magnetic field to stimulate nerve cells in certain areas of the brain. It involves placing a special wand, or magnetic coil, on a precise spot on the scalp. The coil directs magnetic pulses to a portion of the brain involved in mood regulation. Each treatment typically lasts for 40 minutes, five times a week for 4 to 6 weeks, and then is tapered to twice a week for 3 weeks. The dose and position on the scalp are individualized for each person. (The dose, or amount you get, is determined by the strength, pattern, and duration of the magnetic pulse.) Many who have used this treatment have found improvement in their depression symptoms. Other treatments are currently being studied for their effectiveness.

Inpatient Care

Occasionally, someone who has depression is too ill to manage at home or go to outpatient therapy appointments. They may also feel unsafe or suicidal. This situation can overwhelm the person's caretakers. Most people cannot manage this alone.

In this case, they may need treatment in the inpatient psychiatry unit of a hospital. Inpatient care is a more intense form of treatment, where a person receives daily individual and group therapy as well as medication management. An inpatient unit provides a safe environment during a rough time. This is especially important for those who have disorganized or suicidal thoughts.

Once in the hospital, you will be cared for by a treatment team that usually consists of a senior (attending) psychiatrist, nurse, and social worker. If you are in a teaching hospital of a university medical center, you will usually have a psychiatry resident and perhaps a medical student caring for you as well. You may also see a clinical psychologist. The COVID-19 pandemic has somewhat changed the way some of these interactions are done for now.

The inpatient unit will focus on your safety and provide for your daily needs. The treatment team's role is to see you each day, to review your current treatment plan and suggest modifications as required, and to encourage you to attend group therapy sessions with other inpatients. The inpatient treatment plan is a collaborative plan between you and the team. You have the right to decide what feels appropriate and helpful for you and to accept or reject their assessment and recommendations, as long as your decisions are safe.

Most people treated in an inpatient unit find it to be helpful and even lifesaving, although they might not like it very much at the time.

The inpatient team will be in contact with your outpatient providers if you have already established them. If not, the inpatient team will recommend and arrange for a mental health professional, someone who is covered by your insurance plan and located in your area, for you to see following discharge from the hospital. Discharge plans are specific, detailing any changes in medications and treatment plan that you agree to. You will leave the hospital with written instructions and specific appointments already lined up, including what to do if problems arise.

HOW WILL I KNOW IF TREATMENT IS WORKING?

It's good to think about how you might recognize when treatment, including psychotherapy, is effective and working for you. Sometimes you're the last person to notice any improvement in your distressing thoughts, feelings, and behaviors. I urge you to *trust, accept,* and *believe* positive feedback when offered by your family, close friends, and providers.

When you begin treatment, it's most helpful if you set clear goals with your mental health providers. Tell them what is bothering you now, what you would like to change, and in what ways. Share your thoughts on where you'd like to be following treatment. For example, you might say: "I'd like to be less anxious (or sad, or hopeless, or fearful)." "I'd like to have my life back, or at least the parts that were pretty good," or "I'd like to be in a meaningful relationship; finish school; or improve my life in the following way: _____."

You may experience many ups and downs in your emotions during talk therapy and other treatment. Some of this comes from bringing up painful and troubling experiences from your past. Once you've been in treatment for a while, look for small signs of improvement in your life. It doesn't happen immediately and may take some time. Be patient and persistent. You might gradually notice that you've started to reach out to friends more often, making plans for social interactions or things you used to enjoy doing (all before COVID but now done virtually), or have begun to get back into some of your usual work, school, social, and recreational activities. Perhaps you're feeling less irritable and argumentative with your loved ones. Maybe you've stopped drinking or overeating and have started exercising. These are positive signs of improvement. Often, however, you are the last one to notice these subtle differences while it's obvious to your friends and family.

The overall goal in recovery from anxiety, depression, PTSD, or other mental illness, whether or not it's related to the pandemic, is to have a life that is meaningful to you, with purpose and direction, that is based on your own beliefs and convictions, making use of your personal talents and potential, where you will manage life situations well, have positive relationships, and accept yourself. This is what recovery will look like. Trust the process and your mental health team to help direct you to your goals.

WHEN SOMEONE REFUSES TREATMENT

Some people have a hard time accepting treatment for a mental health condition. You may not believe that treatment will help you, may not recognize the need for treatment, or may just plain refuse to go. If you get talked into going, you may go—but unwillingly.

Some people might also reject offers of help from anyone. Families struggle tremendously to convince their loved ones to seek treatment. It is one of the most difficult things people face. Adults have a right to decide for themselves what treatment they receive and what happens to them, including the right to refuse treatment. If you do not perceive the need for treatment, the conversation becomes one sided.

> *NOTE*: A friend or family member cannot force an adult into treatment unless they are in crisis or, in the rare case, legal steps are required to ensure their safety. For example, in the extremely ill, this might mean getting a court order to ensure a person takes their medications. While it's difficult to do, respect their right to refuse your help or treatment unless you believe they could harm themselves or others. Then you must call for professional help or dial 9-1-1 immediately, regardless of the person's preferences.

Reasons for Refusing Treatment

Why would someone who desperately needs treatment refuse it? There are several reasons. You or your loved one may believe that seeking help from a mental health professional means you're a failure. It's hard for someone who has always been able to deal with their own problems to accept help. It may make you feel vulnerable and inadequate. And because of the distorted, negative thinking common in depression, you may perceive any efforts to help as intrusive.

You may be afraid of feeling the strong emotions that treatment may bring up. You may be concerned about the financial burden and paying for treatment. Or your main concern may be privacy issues: you could be afraid that if your friends, coworkers, or employer find out, you will lose your job, reputation, or your friends. You might fear being judged unfairly, criticized, or negatively labeled because of your illness and cut off socially. This is known as the *stigma* of mental illness.

You may also believe that treatment is not effective—at least for you. You may fear becoming dependent on or addicted to medications, dread the side effects they can create, or believe that psychiatric drugs will change who you are. You might also believe the rumors that you will feel like a zombie or lose your creativity on medications. Media reports about the adverse effects of medications and negative television advertisements can also contribute to fears about treatment.

Most of these concerns are based on mistaken beliefs about mental illness and its treatment. The best approach is to learn as much as you can about your illness from reliable sources. Talk to your PCP or someone whose opinion you trust. When misconceptions are cleared up, many people go on to receive effective treatment willingly.

WHAT TO DO IF YOU CANNOT AFFORD MENTAL HEALTH TREATMENT

Health care is expensive. If you live in a country that offers wide-ranging health care coverage, including mental health services, you are fortunate. Despite the foundations of the ACA (Affordable Care Act), more and more people in the United States find they are unable to afford professional mental health services.

Some become unemployed due to the COVID-19 pandemic or their illness and then lose their more comprehensive health care benefits; many others work part time in a job that just does not offer any health care coverage at all. Or there may be insurance limits placed on the number of services a person can receive, thus raising their out-of-pocket expenses. Savings, which are sometimes meager, dwindle. If any of this is true for you, what are your options? Here are a few ideas:

- In-training programs at university teaching hospitals, where clinical care is provided by residents-in-training who are supervised by senior psychiatry staff members
- Sliding-scale clinics where the fee for mental health services is adjusted on a sliding scale for those who have documented financial need
- Pro bono (free) care offered by some mental health professionals—this care depends on the individual provider, and eligibility varies
- School clinics, where mental health care, usually short term, is provided by counselors in high schools and colleges, often for free or at a reduced rate
- Community services, such as mental health clinics offered by state, federal, and local health departments for those in financial need (see a list of resources on the Centers for Disease Control and Prevention (CDC) website, "People Seeking Help," https://www.cdc.gov/mentalhealth/tools -resources/individuals/index.htm).
- Referral to low-cost services through the NAMI (National Alliance on Mental Illness) website (www.NAMI.org) or by calling 800-950-6264
- Listing of mental health facilities provided by SAMHSA (Substance Abuse and Mental Health Services Administration) at "Find Treatment," SAMHSA, https://www .samhsa.gov/find-treatment.

- Employment-based Employee Assistance Programs
  (EAPs) provide mental health services to employees for
  free (for several sessions) or at a reduced rate—check
  with your employer
- The National Suicide Prevention Lifeline at 800-273-8255
  offers emergency assessment

Medications can be expensive, and not all are covered, especially if you have a marginal health insurance plan. There are some ways to get a financial exemption from the pharmaceutical companies (drug manufacturers) for low-cost or free medications for those who meet certain income requirements. You will have to contact each company and apply to them directly if you or your loved one meets their criteria.

CHAPTER 11

Is Talk Therapy Right for Me?

Talk therapy is based on the concept that there is a close connection between our thoughts, feelings, and behaviors (actions). Each of these influences the others. For example, a certain thought may cause you to feel sad. This may then affect your behavior, causing you to cry and withdraw. You then feel even more sadness. Another thought may cause you to feel anxious, and consequently your behavior is jittery.

Talk therapy, or psychotherapy, is a type of guided therapeutic conversation that focuses on this connection, on a person's psychological and emotional problems, distorted thinking, and troublesome behaviors. It can help us cope with our illness, understand ourselves better, acquire the skills and tools to manage stress in healthy ways, make sound life decisions, and adjust to major life losses and transitions. Talk therapy can be done one to one or in a group setting.

COGNITIVE BEHAVIORAL THERAPY

Cognitive behavioral therapy (CBT) is a common and effective type of talk therapy based on the connection between our thoughts, feelings, and actions. CBT teaches a person to identify and change thinking patterns that may be distorted, beliefs that are inaccurate, and behaviors that are unhelpful. You learn to monitor, challenge, and replace your distorted and negative thoughts with more realistic ones and to recognize the link between your thoughts, feelings, and behaviors. This, in turn, will improve how you feel.

Distortions in our thoughts, common in depression and other mental health conditions, are errors in our thinking that twist our interpretation of an event in different ways, oftentimes negative. It could be that we're jumping to conclusions without enough information or the facts behind it; thinking in extremes, such as in a black-and-white, all-or-nothing manner; mind reading what another person is thinking; and in other ways. There is often little or no evidence to support these thoughts. But our interpretations seem true and convincing when we're in the midst of depression. We are more likely to believe the biased or distorted thoughts, even though they are not an accurate reflection of our reality. And we're usually not aware that our thinking is altered in this way, even though these thoughts are extreme and a source of great emotional distress.

It's important to look at whether your thoughts are distorted in some way. One way to do this is to look carefully at

Dr. Thea Gallagher reminds us, "We know if you have a history of a mental health condition, you're more vulnerable when certain life events happen." And yet, many of her patients experiencing anxiety have told her during this time, "I'm glad I have all the tools I learned from therapy." Dr. Gallagher goes on to say that while people with mental health conditions are more vulnerable, people with no skills and tools who've never been to therapy might also struggle with a life transition that they weren't prepared to deal with, thinking "'Oh wow. My whole life changed, and now I need to make sense of that!' It can be difficult for those who might not [have] ever had to think about managing some of their emotional symptoms."

Author interview with Dr. Thea Gallagher, January 15, 2021

the *facts* of a situation and challenge any inaccurate interpretations of them. Thoughts are not facts. Once the distorted thought is replaced with an accurate one, the upsetting emotion will eventually be replaced by a more realistic emotion. This is the basis of CBT, which is particularly useful in depression and anxiety, when our thoughts are often distorted, negative, and upsetting. If we can learn to be more aware of negative and distorted thoughts and feelings and respond to them using CBT, we may be able to avoid a relapse or recurrence of depression or anxiety.

CBT has enduring effects that last beyond the actual treatment period; it is also more likely to prevent recurrence than many other types of therapy.

Many things can make us less accurate in our thinking and interpretation of events, contributing to thought distortions. For example, our thinking can be affected by lack of sleep, poor or imbalanced diet, substance abuse, past experiences, ideas about ourselves and the world (our sense of self-worth), and our mood (such as depression or anxiety). In addition, depression often causes us to view our experiences, ourselves, and our future in a negative, unrealistic way; this is often magnified and may dominate our thinking. The depressed mind tends to interpret and twist things in a down, undesirable direction, causing negative thoughts to happen automatically, not on purpose (they are called *automatic negative thoughts*).

How We Think and Feel Affects How We Act

Normally, we interpret the events in our life and give them meaning; that leads us to have feelings or emotions, such as fear, joy, anger, or sadness. In response to these emotions, we have an urge to act in a certain way. For example, when an event causes us to feel sad and miserable, we may choose to stay in bed, cry, overeat, or drink too much alcohol. While some expression of emotion is okay, these are extreme negative behaviors that are not healthy for us.

Since we have the ability to act on our feelings, we also have some control over our emotions by choosing how we react and respond to them. The actions and decisions we make in response can intensify or lessen a particular feeling. Learning to modify our responses to intense emotion will decrease our level of distress. Cognitive behavioral therapy helps by using a series of exercises to challenge and replace the negative and distorted thoughts that accompany depression and to modify our actions. For example, when using CBT, instead of feeling extremely enraged or out of control in response to a troubling situation, we might feel a little sad or moderately angry and still be able to function. Work with your therapist to learn and practice this skill.

Here's how CBT works. Let's say, for example, that you are upset because a close friend has not returned your phone call or responded to your text message over a few days. You might automatically think, "Oh, he just doesn't like me or care about me." You feel angry and hurt by this, lonely, ignored, and unimportant.

But if you really think about it, this person is a close and loyal friend who has never given you cause for thinking this way—it's an error or distortion in your thinking. So, you might then challenge this negative thought by considering that perhaps they never received your message or had a personal life event that got in the way; maybe they were overwhelmed at school, work, or in their family; or maybe they felt ill.

Acknowledge that you don't really know your friend's reason for delay and replace your automatic thought with something more realistic. For example, you might say to yourself, "John is a close, caring, and trusted friend who has always been there for me and has never just ignored me. There must be a good reason I haven't heard back, and I'll wait to find out. Even though I feel upset now, I'm really more disappointed." Notice that in creating

TABLE 11.1 How to Challenge and Replace Distressing Thoughts

When you recognize that your thinking may be twisted or distorted in some way, CBT skills enable you to challenge these negative and biased thoughts and to replace them with something more accurate. Here's how you do it.

1. Consider a particular situation or event that caused you to feel distress.
2. Identify the negative thought that is automatically raised by this event.
3. Identify the distortions in your thoughts that support your feelings of distress.
4. Notice the emotions you have/had in that moment (sadness, anxiety, fear, etc.).
5. Challenge this negative, distorted thought.
6. Replace the distorted, inaccurate thought with a more realistic alternative thought. The alternative you choose must be a fair and more accurate view of the situation. It has to be realistic, honest, and believable, and it should validate the emotion you are experiencing.
7. Notice the change or improvement in your emotions or in their intensity after you have replaced your negative and distressing thought with a more accurate, realistic view.

this alternative thought around what happened, your emotions have now lifted and you feel moderately disappointed, more understanding, and less intense and negative.

Sometimes the thoughts that bother us come from situations long ago, but these thoughts stay with us even though they no longer apply. Spending time reacting to old thoughts is not productive and doesn't help. One useful CBT exercise is to try understanding where a particular thought comes from, its origin. Ask yourself whether your distressed thought or reaction relates to your current situation or moment or to events from your past.

Does it apply now? If it does not apply now, try to put it aside. Perhaps a certain thought that bothers you began in childhood or adolescence and stems from an unpleasant experience that no longer applies to your current life. It might be something a parent, teacher, or friend said or did that you kept deep inside and that still plagues you now. Sometimes these thoughts stick with us for years, haunting us and causing distress. Spending time reacting to old thoughts that no longer apply is not of value to you in the present.

- Ask yourself: Is your thought or belief inherently true, or is it an internalized message from your past, your environment?
- If it's not true now, try to put it aside
- If you find it is true, think about what is in your power to change.

Another strategy often used in CBT is to look at a troublesome thought and think about the evidence you have in support of or against that thought. The steps to doing this are outlined in table 11.2. The evidence you gather will help you identify and change thoughts that are based on inaccurate assumptions. Use the same compassion in talking to yourself as you would give to others. Doing these exercises often brings relief to those in distress. A summary of different ways to challenge and change your thinking is presented in table 11.3.

Mindfulness-Based CBT

Mindfulness-based CBT is a somewhat different approach that is also effective for some people. The focus is on intentionally being in the moment, not dwelling on past or future events. Mindfulness-based therapy has been found effective in treating depression and anxiety and preventing a recurrence. Please see chapter 2 for more on how to practice mindfulness.

TABLE 11.2 Evidence For and Against

When a thought, belief, or interpretation of an event causes you distress, it's helpful to examine the evidence for and against it. This will help you identify and change thoughts based on inaccurate assumptions.

Step 1. Identify a negative or distressing thought.

Step 2. Gather evidence for and against that thought. List that evidence in the columns below.

- Collect specific evidence or details about the thought to check its accuracy.
- Ask others who know you well for their realistic, honest feedback about the thought.
- Seek out experiences that counteract your negative beliefs. For example, go out and engage in some activity or experience and see if that provides evidence to support, contradict, or disprove your negative belief.

Step 3. Look at your list realistically and see where the evidence lies.

- You will see firsthand that the evidence you gathered most likely speaks against your distressing thought and is not in support of it.

Belief or thought	*Evidence for it*	*Evidence against it*

Source: Susan J. Noonan, *Managing Your Depression: What You Can Do to Feel Better* (Baltimore, MD: Johns Hopkins University Press, 2013), 99–100.

TABLE 11.3 Ways to Challenge and Change Your Thinking

---

1. Look at a situation associated with emotional distress. Identify the distortion in your thought and substitute a more realistic thought or interpretation of that event.

2. Examine the evidence for and against a negative thought, belief, or interpretation of an event (see table 11.2).

3. Examine the pros and cons of any thought, belief, decision, or action.

4. Ask if your belief is inherently true or if it is an internalized message from your environment. If it is true, what is in your power to change?

5. When a thought or belief is upsetting you, look at whether your thought and reaction have more to do with events from long ago. Ask yourself:
   – Where does this thought come from?
   – Does it apply now, in the current situation?

6. Separate your opinion, interpretations, judgments, and emotions from fact. These often distort a situation negatively.
   – Rely on the facts.
   – Ask yourself: Is this an interpretation, a feeling, or is it a fact?

7. Replace *should* statements with less demanding language. Instead of saying, "I should do or be . . ." say "I would like it if . . ."

8. Instead of assuming full responsibility and blame for a particular problem, consider other factors that might have contributed, that were outside your control.

9. Try thinking of things in the middle ground, or gray area, instead of at the extremes of black and white.

DIALECTICAL BEHAVIOR THERAPY

Dialectical behavior therapy (DBT) is another type of psychotherapy. It teaches concrete cognitive behavioral and mindfulness skills in four modules: (1) mindfulness; (2) interpersonal effectiveness, or ways to better manage relationships; (3) emotional regulation, which is helpful in controlling chaotic emotions; and (4) distress tolerance, strategies to get through a difficult time. The skills learned in DBT can help a person deal with issues in a more balanced, less disruptive and irritable manner. DBT has been shown to be an effective additional therapy to antidepressant medication, resulting in improvement in depressive symptoms.

ACCEPTANCE AND COMMITMENT THERAPY

Acceptance and commitment therapy (ACT) is a type of mindfulness-based behavioral therapy that combines mindfulness skills with the practice of self-acceptance. It teaches and encourages people to embrace and accept their distressing thoughts and feelings instead of fighting, struggling with, or avoiding them. ACT helps a person accept what is out of their control, the emotional pain and distress that inevitably accompanies life, and compels them to take action toward reaching their long-term goals, thereby enriching their lives. ACT combined with mindfulness-based therapy is a clinically effective treatment shown to be of benefit in anxiety, depression, and substance use.

EXPOSURE THERAPY

Exposure therapy is a type of talk therapy intervention that helps people face and control their fears and anxiety by carefully and gradually exposing them to the memory and distress of a traumatic or painful situation they have experienced. It's a method to help people break distressing patterns of fear and avoidance, confront those fears, process and deal with the associated emotions, and manage their anxiety. Exposure therapy is done in the context of a safe environment with a trained therapist who is prepared to help you if the exercise brings up distressing emotions. Exposure therapy often uses several different treatment methods, such as mental imagery, writing, or visits to places or people that remind a person of their trauma, anxiety, or distress. When a person is exposed to their unpleasant memories in these ways, over time they are gradually able to become less sensitive and distressed by the feared event. Exposure therapy has been found useful for persons experiencing anxiety, PTSD, prolonged grief disorder, and other mental health conditions.

Sometimes, when the technology is available, exposure therapy is done using a computerized virtual environment that resembles the person's traumatic event (called virtual reality). Like other exposure methods, gradual exposure to the trauma using virtual reality has been a successful treatment in some situations.

BEHAVIORAL ACTIVATION

Loss of interest in the activities a person once enjoyed, which is called anhedonia, is common in depression. This leads people to stop doing those things because they think they are not worth the effort; the depression symptoms worsen, and they feel more isolated, detached, withdrawn, and anxious. Since it's been observed that our behavior affects our emotions and mood in both a positive and a negative way, it's helpful for you to get involved in activities that have the potential to improve your mood, such as doing those things you once enjoyed. This is the basis of behavioral activation, a CBT approach and coping strategy for depression that can positively affect mood, decrease the risk for depression, and help to treat it.

Behavioral activation is a type of behavioral therapy that is often used along with other therapeutic skills and strategies. The aim of behavioral activation is to help a person reengage in enjoyable, rewarding activities and develop or enhance their problem-solving skills. Doing so will counteract the isolation, withdrawal, and avoidance patterns common to depression and in turn improve mood. In addition, doing things that are a little challenging will provide a sense of accomplishment and mastery that may also boost mood.

Behavioral activation is done with a trained therapist who helps you iden-

Behavioral activation is based on getting involved in activities that have the potential to improve your mood.

tify goals (pleasurable activities), schedule positive experiences or activities, address the obstacles to achieving them, and improve problem-solving skills. The goals need to be specific, measurable, attainable, realistic, and trackable.

Dr. Thea Gallagher describes behavioral activation as "more doing" than thinking, in particular doing the things that we normally do that bring us pleasure and enjoyment. Over time that has a very strong impact on how we feel. Behavioral activation conveys, "Your feelings are valid [because] you do feel [a certain] way, but they're not necessarily [an accurate reflection] of how things are. And so, how we're going to combat that is have you do more. You're going to have to do something in the face of how you feel and then see what happens over time. And then ultimately, you'll feel better."

She says that with behavioral activation, you could be unmotivated to do something. You could think, "This is going to stink." But it doesn't matter, and it doesn't matter how you feel after. You just have to move your feet in the direction of doing things in the way that you used to do them when you felt better. The only way to get out of it is that you have to start doing.

Dr. Gallagher recommends that you do behavioral activation in manageable pieces and show your brain through behavior that you can feel different.

Author interview with Dr. Thea Gallagher, January 15, 2021

Once your goals, activities, or positive experiences are identified, you then work to achieve them, striving only for those activities that have personal importance and meaning. Go slow and
start with the easiest ones first, enlisting the support of others
as needed. Behavioral activation can be difficult to do when a
person has low motivation or increased anxiety. This is where
my favorite strategy *action precedes motivation* helps. It means
that you get going and start doing something—an action—even
if you don't feel doing like it right now. The motivation for doing
it will eventually come later.

VIRTUAL VISITS

Social isolation and the COVID-19 pandemic have made access
to mental health professionals challenging. Out of concern for
social distancing during the pandemic, many health care professionals have looked to alternative ways of connecting. Please
refer to chapter 10 for a discussion of virtual visits, or telemedicine.

SUPPORT GROUPS

Often, individuals who receive treatment for depression, anxiety, grief, and PTSD find it helpful to speak with others who are
experiencing the same or similar symptoms. It's a way to realize
that you're not alone in your struggles and allows people to share
problem-solving strategies. Support groups scattered around the
country exist just for this purpose, originally done in person and
now often in virtual support groups because of the pandemic.
The outpatient psychiatry department of a hospital, some community centers, and national patient (consumer) organizations
such as the Depression and Bipolar Support Alliance (DBSA)
or NAMI usually sponsor them. These national organizations

have local chapters and are open to everyone. They also have group sections for friends and family members seeking support. NAMI conducts a training program for families called Family to Family, a 12-week course on accepting and supporting those who have mental illness. More than 300,000 people have taken it so far and have given excellent feedback.

CHAPTER 12

Building and Maintaining Resilience

It's thought that those who cope effectively with the negative effects of stress and their illness may bounce back more readily after an episode of emotional distress, depression, bipolar disorder, anxiety, or other mental illness. This is known as *resilience*, defined by the American Psychological Association (APA) as the "process of adapting well in the face of adversity, trauma, threats, and significant sources of stress—such as family and relationship problems, serious health problems, or workplace and financial stress" (APA 2011).

Think of resilience as an ongoing way of dealing with and navigating through the difficult times in our lives, facing challenges (such as an illness like depression or anxiety or a pandemic), finding solutions, and recovering from setbacks. Having resilience means that you learn effective ways of thinking and responding during difficult situations, including during isolation or a pandemic—you learn from but are not defeated by them. Resilience involves having adaptive behaviors and coping skills, such as problem solving, managing stress, facing one's fears, mastering challenges, regulating one's emotions, and learning the consequences of one's behaviors. These coping strategies can help a person survive and thrive despite hardship.

Resilience is about looking at the situation and our limitations and asking

- What can I do despite these limitations?
- What in my life can I control?

- What are the aspects of this that I can change?
- How can I shift my perspective, adjust my expectations?

Adapting to stress and difficult life events is a complicated process. We learn some of it from our parents and family. It is also likely that genetic factors influence our resilience to adversity. On the other hand, resilience doesn't require a person to have exceptional or unique traits. Rather, it comes from the common inner qualities that surface when we adapt to stress.

When facing a challenge such as the pandemic or social isolation, many people do find a way to cope, to continue on with purposeful lives, even though they may be initially distressed. Finding healthy ways to cope is the foundation of resilience. Yet others find that their distress persists, and they may go on to experience depression or PTSD. Some of this lies in the person's baseline circumstances, skills, opportunities, and differences in emotional, financial, and supportive resources—a lack of such resources makes it more difficult to bounce back from adversity. Some may find that they seem to do well in different areas or phases of their lives and not in others (at work versus home with family stressors; at an older versus younger age). And those who are (temporarily) unable to think clearly or regulate their mood may find it difficult to develop and maintain resilience. For example, this difficulty may happen during an episode of major depression, when the person experiences profound sadness, hopelessness, and clouded thinking.

Resilience involves having hope for recovery and a sense of determination.

You might wonder what makes some people more resilient than others. Southwick and Charney (2012) looked at this very question. They surveyed three groups of people who had experienced extraordinary adversity in life and who survived remarkably well. In the survey responses, they found ten personal characteristics and coping strategies common to those in each of these three groups. They found that people who have resilience used many of these strategies, which they call *resilience factors*. These coping strategies can help a person survive and thrive despite hardship. They are presented for you in table 12.1.

In addition, the APA identifies the following coping strategies (Newman 2002; APA 2011). They are considered important in your efforts to develop resilience, meaning that those who have these traits seem to have an easier time bouncing back from adversity:

- Avoid seeing crises as insurmountable. Develop confidence in your ability to solve problems.
- Accept change as a part of living.
- Form connections with others.
- Make realistic goals and move toward them.
- Take decisive action in difficult situations.
- Look for opportunities for self-discovery.
- Nurture a positive view of yourself.
- Trust your own instincts.
- Keep things in perspective.
- Maintain a hopeful outlook.
- Take care of yourself.
- Maintain flexibility and balance in life.

The APA also notes that caring and supportive relationships, inside and outside the family, are essential to building resilience. They create love and trust, provide role models, and offer encouragement. You'll also see resilience characteristics common to the two lists I just presented to you.

People tend to use various approaches to learn resilience skills. The choice depends on the individual person, the resources they have available through family and friends, and the characteristics of their culture, religion, and community. The culture or community a person was raised in might influence whether and how much they connect with others, communicate

TABLE 12.1 Resilience Factors

1. Maintain an optimistic but realistic outlook.

2. Confront your fears.

3. Rely on your inner core values and altruism.

4. Draw on religious or spiritual practices.

5. Seek and accept social support.

6. Imitate resilient role models.

7. Attend to your physical, mental, and emotional health and well-being.

8. Challenge your mind to maintain brain fitness.

9. Try to maintain cognitive and emotional flexibility—accept that which you cannot change and focus on what you can change.

10. Look for meaning, purpose, and opportunity in the face of adversity.

Source: S. M. Southwick and D. S. Charney, *Resilience: The Science of Mastering Life's Greatest Challenges* (Cambridge: Cambridge University Press, 2012).

their feelings, and deal with adversity. Some people are very private and uncomfortable sharing their feelings, while others reveal every last detail of their emotional life.

If you find yourself temporarily unable to think clearly or are experiencing depression, hopelessness, and lack of energy, you may find it hard to learn the new skills needed to build resilience. Although your overwhelming thinking is often negative, your self-confidence diminished, and your ability to manage strong feelings frequently wanes, these skills aren't impossible to learn. It often just takes the right timing and perseverance.

BUILDING RESILIENCE

Many strategies can help you build resilience, such as those listed below. Don't think that you have to master all of them.

Instead, choose one or two you feel may work and give them a try. If they don't work, or they are too hard to do right now, choose another one or two.

- Seek out *nonjudgmental love and support.*
- Maintain an optimistic but *realistic* outlook. This means holding a reasonable view of the future that involves hope and the confidence that things will turn out well, with enough hard work. Embrace this realistic attitude about your future and try to avoid having unattainable dreams as goals. Focus on what you can do now, with some effort and encouragement. No one can predict the course of anyone's depression or recovery. I've often been reminded that you can never know what's around the corner, what will happen next, whether it's a new treatment for your mental illness disorder or a positive life event.
- Keep an *optimistic attitude* when your emotions fluctuate, which is hard to do. *How?* Try to remember that emotions change and that this situation won't last forever.
- Keep your illness or negative event *in perspective.* Although anxiety or depression is a biological illness that is a part of your life, it does not define you.

Psychologist Dr. Sheila Rauch has found that despite the variability in people's level of resilience, people can be trained to use some skills to help them become more resilient. One thing she has found that predicts a negative mental health response to trauma is the inability of a person to reach out for social supports and to engage with others, feeling more connected. Dr. Rauch has observed that those who are able to access positive social support are more resilient.

Author interview with Dr. Sheila Rauch December 21, 2020

- *Confront your negative thoughts and emotions.* Try to recall past achievements to find evidence for the positive and evidence against the negative views you have of yourself and the world.
- *Recall the inner strengths and resources* you have used to deal with problems in the past. Bring up past successes that obviously show your strengths and abilities. Look for new opportunities to demonstrate those strengths and reinforce your confidence.
- Connect with your *sources of inner strength and joy* (family, friends, pets, music, nature, faith, hobbies). Prioritize relationships.

> *We all have days when we can't face doing these things; they don't click, and none of them seems to work. Be patient and try again tomorrow.*

- *Create concrete and realistic goals.* Plan your future in small, incremental steps. Work to gain the skills to reach your goal, gather the support you need, and take the action to succeed.
- *Learn to face your fears.* Fear can interfere with moving forward and recovering from your illness. It may be helpful if you first accept these fears, gather information about them, and then make plans to confront them. Many people find this far better than passively wishing them away.
- Guide your life by the *core values* you have learned over time and the benefits you have received from reaching out to help others. Core values are the principles, such as honesty, respect, fairness, and compassion, by which we lead our lives. Rely on your inner sense of right and wrong (your moral compass) during periods of stress. Altruism, the act of helping others, and volunteering can bring great benefits as you work to build resilience.

- Consider whether a *spiritual or religious approach* is useful for you. Southwick and Charney (2012) found that some people turn to religion or spirituality to cope with adversity. This approach, they discovered, can lead to lower levels of depression and restore hope and a more balanced view.
- Increase your *social support network*. This is a foundation on which to build resilience. Close supportive relationships build strength and may protect you during stressful times. Isolation and decreased social support frequently lead to increased stress and depression. Find ways to do this during the pandemic.
- Identify a *role model* as a tool to increase your resilience, someone who demonstrates skills and behaviors you may want to imitate. Role models help build resilience through their words and actions. They can help guide a person in learning to manage stress; handle disappointment, difficult life situations, and relationships; make major decisions; and care for themselves physically and emotionally.
- *Take care of your physical and cognitive self* (your mind) and learn self-care. A healthy diet and regular sleep are essential, as is following a daily physical exercise program. Regular exercise acts as an aid to depression and anxiety treatment and lends a sense of self-confidence and self-respect. Physical training helps to improve mood, thinking, self-confidence, and emotional resilience. It also improves mental and emotional health and well-being and decreases the symptoms of depression. Daily brain activity keeps the mind sharp and ready to face life's challenges. Try to read, solve puzzles, or play challenging mind games like Sudoku rather than sit aimlessly on the couch in front of the television.

- *Accept what you cannot change* and focus on what you can do now. Change is a part of living. Accept that certain goals may no longer be attainable as a result of your illness or the pandemic.
- Learn to *control and tolerate strong feelings, emotions, and impulses.* This is frequently done with a therapist, but you can work on it at home.
- Seek a *purpose in life* rather than aimlessly wandering. Find something you enjoy and do well. This might involve taking an educational or training program to achieve new skills. Your purpose could involve school, work, family, sports, social service, or volunteering.
- Build on the *strengths and personal qualities* you already have. Sometimes depression and anxiety make it difficult for a person to see these qualities in themselves.
- Work to *improve your problem-solving skills.*

If you are temporarily unable to think clearly or experience depression, hopelessness, and lack of energy, you may find it hard to learn the new skills needed to build resilience. These skills aren't impossible to learn. It often just takes the right timing and perseverance on your part.

CHAPTER 13

Looking Forward

Reentry Anxiety

The effects of prolonged social isolation or living through events like the COVID-19 pandemic have shaken our sense of well-being and safety. They have led some of us to be fearful of doing anything that might increase our risk of becoming ill or dying, or of infecting or harming our loved ones. Our fears are based on uncertainty and fear of unknown harm, and they are legitimate concerns. In response to this traumatic event, we hunkered down and made major changes in our lives, lifestyles, and behavior. Most of us adopted new and effective routines for our physical and emotional self-care. We've worked from home or assumed the risk as essential workers; homeschooled our children; wore masks; vigorously washed our hands; kept our distance from others; and avoided all but very small social gatherings. Over time we became used to these changes and felt safer in isolation, in a "new normal."

Now that COVID-19 vaccines are available and many communities, cities, states, and nations are working toward reopening, a lot of people feel uneasy about resuming their usual daily life, activities, and behaviors, their "old normal." It's unsettling. A 2021 Stress in America survey conducted by the APA (American Psychological Association) reported that more than 80 percent of people polled experienced emotions associated with prolonged stress, and that about half said they felt uneasy about readjusting to in-person interactions postpandemic. There's apprehension about returning to school, offices, workplaces, shopping centers, restaurants, recreational activities, and social interactions that often include hugs, handshakes, and close physical contact. This apprehension is based on lingering concerns and uncertainty about becoming ill despite vaccination; virus variants; treatment options; the COVID vaccine's long-term effectiveness and side effects, immunity in ourselves, and its safety in our children; the reopening of a "new normal" workplace; and more.

A return to our world following healing from traumatic events is called *reentry*. The emotional experience of reentry is commonly known as *reentry anxiety*, a feeling of excessive worry and nervousness brought on by uncertainty and anticipation of resuming our former way of life following a perceived threat. Anxiety postisolation or postpandemic is related to fear of the unknown, fear of catching or spreading the virus, a feared loss of social interaction skills in some who have fallen out of practice socially during the confinement period, and more. Adding to this, at the time of this writing, anxiety has increased markedly due to a rise in the COVID-19 omicron variant, responsible for illness in both unvaccinated and vaccinated people and resulting in another wave of recommendations and mandates for mask wearing indoors by our infectious disease leadership.

Various anxiety symptoms and experiences within ourselves and in different people are expected and okay. Try to understand that anxiety is a normal reaction to this situation, that a lot of people are feeling this way, and that it will take some effort to manage your anxiety. Also try not to judge yourself or make comparisons to others, as we all experience these events in our own way.

Reentering the world, returning back to a more socially interactive, active, and stimulating life, is often stressful following social isolation or a pandemic. It's hard having to adjust our lives a second time, to turn around and start doing those same things we were just told were dangerous to our health and well-being, especially if our lifestyle changes had been going on a long time or we're fearful or uncertain about how things will go. We're unsure of how to best prepare for a return to in-person activities knowing that some level of risk still continues. We may feel rusty when recruiting our old coping skills, and that drains our confidence in making the transition. It's made more difficult for those of us who are also ex-

Reentry anxiety causes such a degree of worry, fear, and distress that we're often unable to venture out, relax, and enjoy ourselves in public or socially. We think it's not worth the effort.

hausted, burned out, or depressed following social isolation or the pandemic.

Reentry comes with having to adapt to a lot of activities that we're not used to anymore and now find challenging, such as having social interactions all day long; managing resumed family schedules at school and work; negotiating a shopping center or attending a sporting event or religious service; commuting to work; being in traffic; dealing with public transportation; and more. Sometimes there's a negative consequence of reentry, causing us to

- reject invitations to do things that we would have normally accepted before the pandemic
- be unable to relax and enjoy ourselves while out in public because we're still focused on our fears
- believe that socializing isn't worth the amount of anxiety and distress it causes when we do go out
- feel the typical symptoms of anxiety (see chapter 6), such as being lightheaded, jittery, short of breath, nauseated, or sweaty

HOW DO WE MANAGE REENTRY ANXIETY?

First, we must understand that reentry into the world is a gradual process that takes time. Each person should go at their own pace and transition in a way that works for them without feeling pressured by what others think or are doing. The world we live in is now different, with new and evolving rules and expectations, and we're all coming from different isolation and pandemic experiences. Accept that you have a new set of needs and a valid level of discomfort and that it's okay to share them. This means that you decide what boundaries you and your family want to adopt and what activities you are comfortable with. Communicate that to others and then stick with them without feeling guilty or apologetic. For example, you might say, "I've decided to keep more of a distance right now; it's what I'm comfortable doing. I hope you understand," and then leave it at that. Don't try to pressure others to follow you—everyone is entitled to handle things in their own way.

We must base our reentry decisions on reliable information and be prepared to question conflicting statements offered by others or online. Misinformation and ambiguous and ever-changing information circulating at the beginning of the pandemic, and now surrounding vaccinations, has negatively impacted our experience of this illness.

As we face reentry, we must come to terms with what has happened and how it has affected our lives. We must grieve our losses—the loss of loved ones, our health status, lifestyle, employment, opportunities, markers of milestones in life (graduations, weddings, etc.), and financial stability. We may also need to grieve the loss of our prepandemic life and create meaning and understanding for our new normal.

Here's a way to get started. Think about what in your life you have missed that is important to you. Try to imagine practical ways to start living those parts of your life again that were put on hold during isolation or the pandemic. Based on your comfort level, start small and try to slowly face your source(s) of concern and fear. Safely expose yourself to your fears one at a time, allowing yourself time to adjust to the experience, to feel more comfortable with it and less fearful and anxious. Set small goals that will help you get closer to that which you find scary.

For example, you might begin with a grocery store trip, a hike with a few friends, or coffee at a restaurant. Set your mind to expect that it will be enjoyable. Stay in the moment, pay attention to the details, and savor the experience. Then try something else. This is known as *exposure therapy*, a way of safely confronting your sources of fear while working to tolerate them better. Feeling awkward or nervous about doing this does not mean you're doing it wrong—it comes with subjecting yourself to the challenge. Your anxiety should decrease as you put yourself out there more often and begin to adjust.

Another thing that can help is to *manage your level of stress* around your changing and challenging environment. A lower level of overall daily stress enables us to better deal with difficult situations when we're out in public. *How do we do this?* To begin, try to calm your mind when thoughts of pandemic-related threats to your health and safety arise. Remind yourself of the facts and try to develop a tolerance for uncertainty and distress.

Exercising your body and mind is another way to minimize overall stress and anxiety levels. This includes building a combination of regular outdoor walks or other aerobic exercise, muscle relaxation, mindfulness, meditation, stretch, yoga, or deep breathing exercises into your daily routine. It means eating a healthy diet, getting regular sleep, and keeping up with social contacts as discussed in chapter 9. It also means keeping your brain sharp by using it in challenging and creative ways—reading, mind puzzles, playing a musical instrument, learning something new like a new language or craft, and many other ways.

During isolation or the pandemic, you may have spent time doing certain activities or pastimes that you enjoyed and found restful and restorative. Maybe it's playing more with your kids, taking a long walk along a favorite path in your town, gardening, woodworking, or learning a musical instrument. Decide which ones you want to continue doing and how you will fit them into your life going forward; don't just leave it to chance.

Reentry may also be an opportunity for increasing your *resilience*—the ability to rebound after difficult challenges. Resilience means understanding your ability to control a difficult situation and knowing when you must accept and cope with the consequences of what you cannot change. Having or improving your resilience skills will help get you through the anxiety of reentry. This involves accepting change, keeping things in perspective, relying on your inner strengths and core values, making realistic goals, and being flexible. As described in chapter 12, resilience includes having certain adaptive behaviors and skills to solve problems, manage stress and challenges, face our fears, and so forth.

As you face issues around return to your workplace, consider the role that businesses, organizations, and governments play in dealing with various employee experiences and needs. This might include having an employee wellness department that offers education and support, perhaps with regular meetings, where employees feel comfortable confidentially approaching open-minded staff with their concerns and need for stress management and mental health treatment. Decreasing the stigma of mental illness with open, nonjudgmental communication should be a part of this. It might also mean building flexibility into the schedule and work model to accommodate employee needs, prioritize self-care, encourage taking breaks and allotted vacation time, and perhaps implementing a policy to limit expectations on response to email to the standard working hours of the organization. The University of California at San Francisco (UCSF) Employee Coping and Resiliency Program has some tips for managers to support employees who may feel anxious about returning to in-person work. It can be found at "Re-Entering the Workplace: A Manager's Guide," https://psychiatry.ucsf.edu/sites /psych.ucsf.edu/files/Cope%20Re-Entry%20Guide%20for%20 Managers.pdf.

WHEN TO SEEK PROFESSIONAL HELP

Many people will be able to deal with their anxiety and make the transition to a satisfactory postisolation or postpandemic life on their own, using the self-help recommendations described in this book. If your symptoms of anxiety during reentry become excessive and interfere with your ability to function in one or more areas of your life, however, it's time to seek professional help. For example, perhaps you are unable to leave your home, do your work, or maintain relationships with your friends and family; find yourself continually cleaning with disinfectant or excessively washing your hands; or you've become preoccupied with fears of getting sick. These are signs that you're not managing your postpandemic anxiety very well. A therapist or other mental health provider can help you get through this time. You might wonder how.

Mental health professionals can help you understand yourself better, learn healthy ways to cope and manage stress, make sound life decisions, and adjust to major losses and life transitions. They can help you move through reentry by helping you face your fear and anxiety, deal with loss and grief, build resilience, polish your coping skills, overcome pandemic fatigue, enable you to help your children return to school and their active lives, and in many other ways. While most of this is done in talk therapy, medications are often effectively used to help you deal with symptoms of stress, anxiety, prolonged grief, PTSD, or depression.

This book covers more information on stress and coping skills in chapter 2, facing our fears in chapter 3, understanding and dealing with anxiety in chapter 6, and cultivating resilience in chapter 12. I encourage the reader to review these sections again as needed.

Final Thoughts

Here, I'd like to share with you some thoughts I have on mental illness and its treatment. The widespread occurrence of depression, anxiety, and other mental health conditions during periods of social isolation, such as during the COVID-19 pandemic, tells us that we are not alone in this and that there is no shame in experiencing a mental illness. We must not be afraid to seek professional mental health care. In addition, we must continue to improve the way society and all professions regard depression, anxiety, PTSD, and other mental illnesses. Our role as persons who have lived experience with a mental illness is to inspire new thinking and a change in attitude in professional, academic, and private settings. To inspire such, here are several steps we can take to make a positive impact. Addressing these issues will do a lot to decrease stigma and encourage mental health treatment for all.

1. Understand that stigma is based on misinformation, fear, and arrogance. Continued education about mental illness as well as effective treatment options is key.
2. Policy change around mental health care and access is needed on an institutional level. Our work, academic, community, and religious institutions need to openly discuss mental health conditions as treatable biological illnesses and offer time and resources for treatment. These changes need to be comprehensive, meaningful, and adhered to, and they must translate well within our environments. When this message comes from the top, others are more likely to accept it.
3. Building on these educational efforts and policy changes, a cultural shift in the way mental illness is regarded

needs to occur. This is most effective when it trickles down from leadership in our organizations, schools, communities, and other social structures. Creating an environment that encourages openness and wellness, and dispels fear of disclosure, is the minimum prerequisite.

4. We all need to be open and nonjudgmental, talking about mental illness and the treatments involved freely and in a compassionate way. This will go far in dispelling the stigma and fears around it.

Psychoeducation and policy improvements are not enough to accomplish lasting change. It is essential that those who have lived experience share their stories. When friends, classmates, neighbors, and colleagues who have successfully received help for depression, anxiety, suicidality, PTSD, and other mental illness share their experiences, without fear of repercussion, more of us in need of psychiatric treatment will feel comfortable seeking and receiving appropriate care.

Glossary

anxiety. A feeling of excessive nervousness, apprehension, and worry about the future; the depth of worry, length of time it lasts, and how often it occurs is out of proportion to the actual event.

automatic negative thoughts. Thoughts that occur quickly and involuntarily during episodes of depression that cause distress. They arise because (1) negative events dominate the thinking of someone who has depression, and (2) the depressed mind tends to interpret and twist things in a negative direction. These thoughts don't accurately reflect reality.

behavioral activation. A CBT skill and coping strategy for depression that can positively impact mood, decrease the risk for depression, and help treat it. The aim of behavioral activation is to help a person reengage in enjoyable, rewarding activities and develop or enhance their problem-solving skills.

bipolar depression. A biologically based illness that negatively affects one's thoughts, emotions, and behaviors. It is relapsing and remitting yet treatable and alternates with episodes of extreme elevated mood (mania or hypomania). It affects relationships, activities, interests, and many other aspects of life. Bipolar depression is thought to involve a dysfunction of the network of *neurons* (brain cells) in the brain.

bipolar disorder. A biologically based illness with a major impact on daily life. Also known as *manic-depressive disorder*, it is thought to result from a dysfunction of the network of neurons in the brain. Bipolar disorder is characterized by episodes of extreme elevated mood or irritability (mania or hypomania) followed by episodes of depression.

boundaries. Rules or limits on behavior that are agreed on by
you and another person.

burnout. The sense of having reached the limits of your
endurance and your ability to cope with a situation. Burnout is the result of too many demands on your strength,
resources, time, and energy.

cognitive behavioral therapy (CBT). A kind of talk therapy, or
psychotherapy, that addresses the connection between our
thoughts, feelings, and actions. CBT teaches a person to
identify and change thinking patterns that may be distorted, beliefs that are inaccurate, and behaviors that are
unhelpful.

cognitive distortions. Errors in thinking that twist a person's
interpretation of an event. This is common in depression.
CBT uses exercises to challenge and replace the negative
and distorted thoughts with more realistic thoughts.

coping strategies. The things we do to ease the stressors and
challenges of daily life. Coping includes problem solving,
self-soothing, relaxation, distraction, humor, mindfulness
meditation, and other techniques.

depression. A biologically based illness that negatively affects
one's thoughts, emotions, and behaviors. Depression is a
relapsing and remitting yet treatable illness of the mind
and body. It affects relationships, activities, interests, and
many other aspects of life. Depression is thought to involve a dysfunction of the network of neurons in the brain.
This may happen when certain life experiences occur in a
susceptible person.

difficult-to-treat depression (DTD). A way to describe the
condition of those who do not respond to treatment after
repeated efforts. DTD involves a shift away from a goal of
complete remission to one of optimal symptom control
and functional improvement, where the inconvenience,

side effects, and burden of repeated treatments on patients' lives are minimized.

distorted thinking. Errors in thinking that twist someone's
interpretation of an event. CBT uses a series of exercises to
challenge and replace the negative and distorted thoughts
that accompany depression.

dual diagnosis. A term that describes those who experience
a mental illness and a substance use disorder at the same
time.

DSM-5. The *Diagnostic and Statistical Manual of Mental Disorders*, 5th edition, is published by the American Psychiatric
Association as the standard manual used by mental health
professionals to identify the symptoms and criteria used
in diagnosing mental illness.

essential worker. A person who continues to work to provide
necessary services in times of disaster, emergency, or difficult circumstances, such as during a pandemic: health care
workers, first responders, fire and police, clerks in grocery
stores and pharmacies, maintenance and utility workers,
and so forth.

exposure therapy. A type of talk therapy that helps people
face and control their fears and anxiety by gradually and
carefully exposing them to the memory and distress of a
traumatic or painful situation they experienced.

gene × environment. A theory of depression that involves
the interaction of our genes and the events in our life
(our environment), which shape the complex network of
cells in the brain.

grief. The natural psychological reaction to the loss of someone or something you love.

hypomania. An elevated, hyper mood that is part of bipolar I
disorder. It comes in episodes that alternate with *bipolar
depression*, and the pattern is unique to each person. The

symptoms are similar to mania. Hypomania is of shorter
duration and less intense than mania.

impairment (functional). A decrease in a person's ability to
perform the normal daily activities of life (including work,
school, family, social, recreational).

loneliness. An overwhelming sense of being cut off and apart
from others, regardless of who or how many people are
included in our social circle or home life. It is the gap
between the social connections we desire and what we
actually experience.

major depression. A treatable, biologically based illness that
negatively affects one's thoughts, feelings, and behaviors. Depression is a relapsing and remitting illness of the
mind and body. It affects relationships, activities, interests,
and various other aspects of life. Depression is thought
to involve a dysfunction of the network of neurons in the
brain. This may happen when certain life experiences
occur in a susceptible person.

mania. An elevated, hyper mood that is part of bipolar II
disorder. It comes in episodes unique to each person and
alternates with bipolar depression. The symptoms of elevated mood affect our thoughts, feelings, and behaviors.
They include an inflated sense of self, increased physical
energy, a decreased need for sleep, racing thoughts, irritability, high-risk behaviors, and others.

metabolic syndrome. A physical condition that consists of
having three of the following five cardiovascular risk
factors: central (around the midsection) obesity, high
blood pressure, high levels of triglycerides (fat) in the
blood, low levels of the "good" HDL cholesterol, or high
levels of fasting blood sugar. Having metabolic syndrome
puts you at increased chance of having a heart attack,
stroke, or diabetes.

mindfulness. A way of living your life by focusing on the present moment, on purpose and nonjudgmentally. You pay attention to *now* and avoid ruminating about the past or worrying about the future.

mood disorders. Conditions of the brain that involve the state of mind—the part of our inner self that colors and drives thoughts, feelings, and behaviors. Mood disorders are treatable biological illnesses. Mood disorders include major depression and bipolar disorder.

pandemic. The spread to more than one continent of an infectious disease to which people do not have immunity.

postpartum depression. Tearfulness, sadness, varying moods, irritability, and anxiety that peaks 2–5 days after childbirth and lasts about 2 weeks. It may be mild or deep and extreme and impairs functioning and the infant-caregiver attachment. Postpartum depression is related to a rapid shift in hormones experienced by the woman.

post-traumatic growth (PTG). The positive (psychological) life changes that sometimes happen following a stressful, upsetting, or highly challenging experience.

post-traumatic stress disorder (PTSD). A severe, disabling mental health disorder that sometimes occurs after exposure to a traumatic event. It includes distressing memories, nightmares, flashbacks, hypervigilance, hyperarousal, and avoidance behaviors.

primary care physician (PCP). Such as a person's family doctor, pediatrician, or internist.

prolonged grief response. When grief is persistent, with emotional distress and impaired functioning.

psychotherapy. Talk therapy, a type of guided therapeutic conversation that focuses on a person's psychological and emotional problems, distorted thinking, and troublesome behaviors. It can help you cope with your illness, understand yourself better, learn healthy ways to manage stress, make sound life decisions, and adjust to major life losses and transitions.

realistic optimism. A reasonable view of the future that involves hope and the confidence that things will turn out well, with enough hard work and determination.

recovery. A process of change through which individuals improve their health and wellness, live a self-directed life, and strive to reach their full potential. Recovery is an ongoing process of gaining control of your life after a psychiatric diagnosis and all of the losses that accompany it.

recurrence. The return of full depressive symptoms following a *full recovery* from an episode.

relapse. The return of full depressive symptoms after *partial recovery* from an episode.

remission. Depressive symptoms completely cleared.

resilience. The ability to face adversity and challenges (such as an illness like depression or bipolar disorder, social isolation, or a pandemic), find solutions, and recover from setbacks.

resilience factors. A set of characteristics common to those who adapt well to stressful times.

response. Partial improvement in symptoms and at least a 50 percent reduction in depression severity as measured by standardized rating questionnaires.

shared decision making. A process in which you or your loved one and the clinician work together to make decisions and select diagnostic tests, treatments, and care plans based on clinical evidence while balancing the risks and benefits with personal preferences and values.

sleep hygiene. The personal habits, behaviors, and environmental conditions that affect a person's sleep. These include going to bed and waking up at the same time seven days a week, reserving the bed for sleep only, avoiding caffeine after noon, and more. These habits have a positive impact on the quality and quantity of sleep.

social distancing. The public health mandate to keep a specific distance apart from another person, usually for safety reasons; in the case of COVID-19, we are required to keep 6 feet apart from each other and have no more than ten people gather together indoors (at a restaurant table, for example).

social isolation. Physical and social separation from other people.

solitude. Restorative time spent alone, by choice, which has a purpose and is often soothing and rejuvenating.

somatic therapy. Those treatments that are physically applied to the body and have an effect on the brain, for example, electroconvulsive therapy, transcranial magnetic stimulation, and others.

stigma. An unfounded, hurtful, and unfair negative label or critical judgment placed on a person because of a mental illness; stigma may lead to being avoided, rejected, or shunned by others.

stress. An emotionally and physically disturbing condition you may have in response to changing and challenging life events.

suicide, risk factors for. A set of personal life history conditions or events that may make it more likely that a person will take their life.

suicide, warning signs. A set of behaviors that may indicate a person is contemplating harming themselves or taking their own life.

support. The time spent listening, hearing, and acknowledging the emotions that someone is experiencing. It also includes advocating on their behalf.

telehealth. A general term for a broad array of technologies and tactics that deliver virtual medical visits as well as other health services and health education.

telemedicine. Medical or mental health appointments done virtually on a computer or telephone.

treatment-resistant depression (TRD). The failure to respond or achieve remission after an adequate course of acceptable treatment of an antidepressant or other treatment, in a standard dose and duration (one or three or more courses of treatment—this is not yet specified).

triggers. Events or circumstances that may cause someone distress and lead to an increase in symptoms of depression, post-traumatic stress disorder, or other mental illness.

virtual appointments. Medical or mental health appointments done virtually on a computer or telephone; also known as *telemedicine.*

warning signs of depression. Distinct changes from a person's usual thoughts, feelings, behaviors, routine, or self-care noticed by others. These changes may indicate a new or worsening episode of depression.

well-being. Having a sense of realizing your full potential, with improvement over time, with positive relationships, a feeling of independence and being in control of your life, a sense of competence and mastery, and feeling good about yourself.

Zoom fatigue. A state of extreme tiredness, worry, or burnout associated with overusing technology for virtual communication.

Resources

SOME OF THE MANY BOOKS THAT MAY BE OF INTEREST

Herbert Benson. *The Relaxation Response.* Avon; 1975, 2000.

Norman T. Berlinger. *Rescuing Your Teenager from Depression.* HarperCollins; 2006.

David B. Burns. *Feeling Good: The New Mood Therapy.* Harper-Collins; 2009.

Nell Casey. *Unholy Ghost: Writers on Depression.* William Morrow; 2001.

Adele Faber and Elaine Mazlish. *How to Talk So Teens Will Listen and Listen So Teens Will Talk.* William Morrow; 2005.

Roger Fisher and William Ury. *Getting to Yes: Negotiating Agreement without Giving In.* Penguin; 1983, 1991, 2012.

Felice Jacka. *Brain Changer: The Good Mental Health Diet.* Macmillan Australia; 2019.

Kay Redfield Jameson. *An Unquiet Mind: A Memoir of Mood and Madness.* Vintage Books (Random House); 1995.

Jon Kabat-Zinn. *Wherever You Go, There You Are: Mindfulness Meditation in Everyday Life.* Hyperion; 1994.

Elisabeth Kübler-Ross. *On Death and Dying.* Simon & Schuster; 1969, 2014.

Elisabeth Kübler-Ross and David Kessler. *On Grief and Grieving: Finding the Meaning of Grief through the Five Stages of Loss.* Scribner; 2014.

David J. Miklowitz. *The Bipolar Disorder Survival Guide: What You and Your Family Need to Know.* 3rd ed. Guilford Press; 2019.

Francis Mark Mondimore. *Bipolar Disorder: A Guide for You and Your Loved Ones.* 4th ed. Johns Hopkins University Press; 2020.

Francis Mark Mondimore. *Depression, the Mood Disease.* 3rd ed. Johns Hopkins University Press; 2006.

Francis Mark Mondimore and Patrick Kelly. *Adolescent Depression: A Guide for Parents.* 2nd ed. Johns Hopkins University Press; 2015.

Vivek H. Murthy. *Together: The Healing Power of Human Connection in a Sometimes Lonely World.* HarperCollins; 2020.

Susan J Noonan. *Helping Others with Depression: Words to Say, Things to Do.* Johns Hopkins University Press; 2020.

Susan J. Noonan. *Managing Your Depression: What You Can Do to Feel Better.* Johns Hopkins University Press; 2013.

Susan J. Noonan. *Take Control of Your Depression: Strategies to Help You Feel Better Now.* Johns Hopkins University Press; 2018.

John J. Ratey with Eric Hagerman. *Spark: The Revolutionary New Science of Exercise and the Brain.* Little, Brown; 2008.

Laura Epstein Rosen and Xavier F. Amador. *When Someone You Love Is Depressed: How to Help Your Loved One without Losing Yourself.* Fireside / Simon & Schuster; 1996.

Deborah Sichel and Jeanne Watson Driscoll. *Women's Moods: What Every Woman Must Know about Hormones, the Brain, and Emotional Health.* Quill; 1999.

Andrew Solomon. *The Noonday Demon: An Atlas of Depression.* Scribner; 2001.

Steven M. Southwick and Dennis S. Charney. *Resilience: The Science of Mastering Life's Greatest Challenges.* Cambridge University Press; 2012.

William Styron. *Darkness Visible: A Memoir of Madness.* Vintage Books; 1990.

William Ury. *Getting Past No: Negotiating in Difficult Situations.* Bantam; 1993, 2007.

Mark Williams, John Teasdale, Zindel Segal, and Jon Kabat-Zinn. *The Mindful Way through Depression: Freeing Yourself from Chronic Unhappiness.* Guilford Press; 2007.

ORGANIZATIONS THAT MAY BE OF INTEREST

American Foundation for Suicide Prevention (AFSP)
https://afsp.org

The AFSP funds research, provides educational programs for professionals, and educates the public about mood disorders and suicide prevention. It also promotes policies and legislation on suicide prevention and provides resources for survivors of suicide loss and people at risk.

Anxiety and Depression Association of America (ADAA)
https://adaa.org

ADAA is an international nonprofit membership organization providing education, training, and research for anxiety, depression, and related disorders. Log on to find current treatment and research information and to access free resources and support.

Beyond Blue
www.beyondblue.org.au

This website of the National Depression Initiative of Australia contains information for those with depression, anxiety, and suicide risk. Support comes in the form of telephone and online chat, email, and online forums.

College Suicide Prevention

www.affordablecollegesonline.org/college-resource-center/college-suicide-prevention

This guide was designed to offer hope and help for those who are experiencing suicidal thoughts, as well as the friends and family who want so badly to help them.

Depression and Bipolar Support Alliance (DBSA)

www.dbsalliance.org

The DBSA's mission is to provide "hope, help, support, and education to improve the lives of people who have mood disorders." The DBSA has local chapters with support groups that meet regularly, national educational meetings, online wellness tools, an advocacy center, and training programs for peer specialists. You can share ideas in its online community, the Facing Us Clubhouse.

Depression and Bipolar Support Alliance (DBSA) Balanced Mind Parent Network

www.dbsalliance.org/support/for-friends-family/for-parents/balanced-mind-parent-network/

This is a program of the DBSA to guide families raising children with mood disorders to get the answers, support, and stability they seek.

Families for Depression Awareness

www.familyaware.org

A national organization in the United States to help families recognize and cope with depression and bipolar disorder, get people well, and prevent suicides.

International Bipolar Foundation (IBPF)

https://ibpf.org

The goal of the IBPF is to improve the understanding and treatment of bipolar disorder through research, to promote care and support resources for individuals and caregivers, and to erase stigma through education.

Man Therapy

https://mantherapy.org

Using humor to show working-age men that talking about their problems and getting help is not a sign of weakness, Man Therapy provides men, and the people who care about them, information and resources about men's mental health. They cover how to recognize signs and physical manifestations of stress, examine their own wellness, and connect with resources.

McMan's Depression and Bipolar Web

www.mcmanweb.com

This is a great website on depression and bipolar disorder run by John McManamy, an award-winning journalist and author who has bipolar illness.

National Alliance for Mental Illness (NAMI)

www.nami.org

NAMI is the largest grassroots mental health organization in the United States. It provides information about mental illness, treatment options, support groups, and programs. You can go online to find a link to your local NAMI chapter. NAMI runs a highly regarded training program called Family to Family, a 12-week evidence-based course on accepting and supporting those with mental illness. Approximately 300,000 people have completed it.

National Center for PTSD

www.ptsd.va.gov

A national center for PTSD education and support. They also provide self-help, education, and support apps for PTSD, mindfulness, insomnia (including CBT-I), and other areas. (For the mobile apps, see www.ptsd.va.gov/appvid/mobile/index.asp.)

National Institute of Mental Health (NIMH)

www.nimh.nih.gov

This national organization supports research on mental illness and provides information about depression and bipolar disorder, including current research and clinical trials.

Now Matters Now

www.nowmattersnow.org

This site offers tools for coping with suicidal thoughts, direct easy-to-follow videos, as well as strategies to help those who have depression build more manageable and meaningful lives. As it was developed by Marsha Linehan, PhD, creator of dialectical behavior therapy (DBT), it focuses on techniques such as mindfulness and paced breathing.

Psych Education

https://psycheducation.org

This is an educational website run by Jim Phelps, MD, an active clinician and author with expertise in bipolar disorder and depression.

Support for College Students with Bipolar Disorder

www.affordablecollegesonline.org/college-resource-center/college-student-bipolar-disorder

This guide focuses on how students with bipolar disorder can find help on campus, the importance of continuing treatment plans, and how to make the college experience both a success and a wonderful time.

This Is My Brave

https://thisismybrave.org

Their mission is to end the stigma of mental illness by sharing personal stories of people overcoming mental illness through poetry, essays, original music, live stage performance, stories published to their blog, and YouTube videos.

ONLINE INFORMATION THAT MAY BE OF INTEREST

American Psychological Association (APA), "Building Your Resilience"

www.apa.org/topics/resilience

This online brochure defines *resilience* as the "process of adapting well in the face of adversity, trauma, threats, and significant sources of stress—such as family and relationship problems, serious health problems, or workplace and financial stress." It provides personal strategies for developing and enhancing resilience.

Dietary Guidelines for Americans, 2020–2025

www.dietaryguidelines.gov/sites/default/files/2020-12
/Dietary_Guidelines_for_Americans_2020-2025.pdf

This is the latest US Department of Agriculture (USDA) diet and nutritional guidance for all Americans. It includes information on nutrients and their health benefits, portion sizes, weight management and calories, daily food plans, nutrition during pregnancy, and physical activity. Interactive tools are available at the USDA My Plate website: www.myplate.gov.

Mental Health First Aid (MHFA)

www.mentalhealthfirstaid.org

MHFA is an international program currently active in 24 countries that teaches the skills to respond to the signs of mental illness and substance use. The 2016 guidelines for how to talk to someone who is suicidal can be found at the Australian MHFA website at https://mhfa.com.au/sites/default/files /MHFA_suicide_guidelinesA4%202014%20Revised.pdf.

MGH Center for Women's Mental Health

www.womensmentalhealth.org

This online library of articles, a blog, and newsletters sponsored by the Department of Psychiatry of the Massachusetts General Hospital (MGH) provides the latest information on mental health for women in all stages of life. The focus is primarily on mood disorders during the reproductive (childbearing) and menopausal years. There are also links to both the Clinical Program and the Research Program at the MGH Center for Women's Mental Health.

Physical Activity Guidelines for Americans, 2nd edition

https://health.gov/paguidelines/second-edition/pdf/Physical _Activity_Guidelines_2nd_edition.pdf

This PDF contains guidelines on how much exercise you need at every age, how to add physical activity to your life, and how to measure the intensity of your physical exercise session.

ONLINE TOOLS THAT MAY BE OF INTEREST

COVID Coach App

www.ptsd.va.gov/appvid/mobile/COVID_coach_app.asp

COVID Coach is a free, easy-to-use, evidence-based mobile app from the VA National Center for PTSD, with self-care strategies designed to promote health and wellness for anyone affected by the COVID-19 pandemic. The app, available for Apple and Android devices, includes brief, simple tools and resources for coping, mindfulness, stress, sleep, mood, and anxiety management and wellness.

The Scientific 7 Minute Workout

https://www.nytimes.com/interactive/projects/well/workouts/

New York Times author Gretchen Reynolds provides a set of comprehensive yet quick physical exercises that you can do anywhere.

References

Specia M. Print edition: Their community in crisis: Fishermen answer call. *New York Times*, Dec. 7, 2020, Section A, page 4. Online edition: As pandemic threatens Britain's mental health, these "Fishermen" fight back. NY Times, 2020. https://www.nytimes.com/2020/12/06 /world/europe/uk-mental-health-suicide-coronavirus.html?action =click&campaign_id=154&emc=edit_cb_20201207&instance_id =24804&module=RelatedLinks&nl=coronavirus-briefing&pgtype =Article&regi_id=20178557&segment_id=46290&te=1&user_id =dcaf0551c2a6a11f089a1273716ef107. Accessed December 2020.

Introduction and Chapter 1. What Is Social Isolation?

Ahmed H, Patel K, Greenwood D, et al. 2020. Long-term clinical outcomes in survivors of severe acute respiratory syndrome (SARS) and Middle East respiratory syndrome coronavirus (MERS) outbreaks after hospitalization or ICU admission: A systematic review and meta-analysis. *J Rehabil Med.* 52(5):1–11. DOI:10.2340/16501977-2694.

Alcaraz KI, Eddens KS, Blasé JL, et al. 2019. Social isolation and mortality in US Black and white men and women. *Am J Epidemiol* 188(1): 102–9.

Bernstein E, Blunden H, Brodsky A, Sohn W, Waber B. 2020. The implications of working without an office. *Harvard Bus Rev*, July 15, 2020. https://hbr.org/2020/07/the-implications-of-working-without-an-office.

Beutel ME, Klein EM, Brahler E, et al. 2017. Loneliness in the general population: Prevalence, determinants and relations to mental health. *BMC Psychiatry* 17:97. DOI:10.1186/s12888-017-1262-x.

Brooks SK, Webster RK, Smith LE, et al. 2020. The psychological impact of quarantine and how to reduce it: Rapid review of the evidence. *Lancet* 395(10227):912–20. https://doi.org/10.1016/S0140-6736(20) 30460-8.

Byambasuren O, Cardona M, Bell K, et al. 2020. Estimating the extent of asymptomatic COVID-19 and its potential for community transmission: Systematic review and meta-analysis. *JAAMI* 5(4):223-34. https:// doi.org/10.3138/jammi-2020-0030.

Cacioppo JT, Hughes ME, Waite LJ, et al. 2006. Loneliness as a specific risk factor for depressive symptoms: Cross-sectional and longitudinal analyses. *Psychology and Aging* 21(1):140–51. https://doi.org/10.1037/0882-7974.21.1.140.

Callahan M. "Zoom fatigue" is real: Here's why you're feeling it, and what you can do about it. *News @ Northeastern*, May 11, 2020. https://news .northeastern.edu/2020/05/11/zoom-fatigue-is-real-heres-why-youre -feeling-it-and-what-you-can-do-about-it/.

Calls to suicide and help hotline in Los Angeles increase 8,000% due to coronavirus. Eyewitness News 7 ABC (KABC), Los Angeles, CA, April 20, 2020. https://abc7.com/suicide-hotline-calls-coronavirus-covid19 -los-angeles/6117099/.

Centers for Disease Control and Prevention (CDC). 2017. Quarantine and isolation. Last reviewed Sept. 29, 2017. https://www.cdc.gov/quarantine /index.html.

Centers for Disease Control and Prevention (CDC). 2021a. Anxiety and depression: Household pulse survey. Last reviewed Oct. 20, 2021. https://www.cdc.gov/nchs/covid19/pulse/mental-health.htm.

Centers for Disease Control and Prevention (CDC). 2021b. Scientific brief: SARS-CoV-2 transmission. Updated May 7, 2021. https:www.cdc.gov /coronavirus/2019-ncov/more/scientific-brief-sars-cov-2.html.

Centers for Disease Control and Prevention (CDC). 2021c. Understanding how COVID-19 vaccines work. Updated May 27, 2021. https://www .cdc.gov/coronavirus/2019-ncov/vaccines/different-vaccines/how-they -work.html.

Chopra V, Flanders SA, O'Malley M, et al. 2021. Sixty-day outcomes among patients hospitalized with COVID-19. *Ann Int Med* 174(4): 576–78. https://doi.org/10.7326/M20-5661.

Cigna. 2018. Cigna U.S. loneliness index: Survey of 20,000 Americans examining behaviors driving loneliness in the United States. May 2018. https://www.cigna.com/assets/docs/newsroom/loneliness-survey-2018 -full-report.pdf

Cigna. 2020. *Loneliness and the Workplace: 2020 U.S. Report.* https:// www.cigna.com/static/www-cigna-com/docs/about-us/newsroom /studies-and-reports/combatting-loneliness/cigna-2020-loneliness -factsheet.pdf.

Covid-19 Mental Disorders Collaborators. 2021. Global prevalence and burden of depressive and anxiety disorders in 204 countries and territories in 2020 due to the COVID-19 pandemic. *Lancet.* Published online October 8, 2021. https://doi.org/10.1016/S0140-6736(21)02143-7.

Cutler DM, Summers LH. 2020. The COVID-19 pandemic and the $16 trillion virus. *JAMA* 324(15):1495–96.

Czeisler MÉ, Lane RI, Petrosky E, et al. 2020. Mental health, substance use, and suicidal ideation during the COVID-19 pandemic—United States, June 24–30, 2020. *MMWR Morb Mortal Wkly Rep* 69:1049–57. http://dx.doi.org/10.15585/mmwr.mm6932a1.

del Rio C, Collins LF, Malani P. 2020. Long-term health consequences of COVID-19. *JAMA* 324(17):1723–24. DOI:10.1001/jama.2020.19719.

Donovan NJ, WU Q, Rentz DM, et al. 2017. Loneliness, depression and cognitive function in older U.S. adults. *Int J Geriatr Psychiatry* 32(5): 564–73. DOI:10.1002/gps.4495.

Ettman CK, Abdalla SM, Cohen GH, et al. 2020. Prevalence of depression symptoms in US adults before and during the COVID-19 pandemic. *JAMA Network Open* 3(9):e2019686. DOI:10.1001/jamanetworkopen .2020.19686.

Evans ML, Lindauer M, Farrell ME. 2020. A pandemic within a pandemic—Intimate partner violence during COVID-19. *N Engl J Med* 383(24):2302–4.

Fitzpatrick KM, Drawve G, Harris C. 2020. Facing new fears during the COVID-19 pandemic: The state of America's mental health. *J Anxiety Disord* 75:102291. DOI:10.1016/j.janxdis.2020.102291.

Frank E. 2007. Interpersonal and social rhythm therapy: A means of improving depression and preventing relapse in bipolar disorder. *J Clin Psychology: In Session* 63(5):463–73.

Galea S, Merchant RM, Lurie N. 2020. The mental health consequences of COVID-19 and physical distancing: The need for prevention and early intervention. *JAMA Int Med* 180(6):817–18. DOI:10.1001/jama internmed.2020.1562.

Hawkley LC, Cacioppo JT. 2010. Loneliness matters: A theoretical and empirical review of consequences and mechanisms. *Ann Behav Med* 40(2):218–27. DOI:10.1007/s12160-010-9210-8.

Hawkley LC, Capitanio J. 2015. Perceived social isolation, evolutionary fitness and health outcomes: A lifespan approach. *Phil Trans R Soc B* 370:20140114. http://dx.doi.org/10.1098/rstb.2014.0114.

Hawkley LC, Thisted RA, Cacioppo JT. 2009. Loneliness predicts reduced physical activity: Cross-sectional and longitudinal analysis. *Health Psychol* 28(3):354–63. DOI:10.1037/a0014400.

Hawryluck L, Gold WL, Robinson S, et al. 2004. SARS control and psychological effects of quarantine, Toronto, Canada. *Emerg Infect Dis* 10(7):1206–12. DOI:10.3201/eid1007.030703.

Holt-Lunstad J, Smith TB, Baker M, et al. 2015. Loneliness and social isolation as risk factors for mortality: A meta-analytic review. *Perspect Psychol Sci* 10(2):227–37. DOI:10.1177u/1745691614568352.

Johansson MA, Quandelacy TM, Kada S, et al. 2021. SARS-CoV-2 transmission from people without COVID-19 symptoms. *JAMA Network
Open* 4(1):e2035057. DOI:10.1001/jamanetworkopen.2020.35057.

Klass P. 2020. What pediatricians say can't wait. *New York Times*, Dec.
21, 2020. https://www.nytimes.com/2020/12/21/well/family/children
-health-pandemic.html.

Lee AM, Wong, JGWS, McAloan GM, et al. 2007. Stress and psychological distress among SARS survivors 1 year after the outbreak.
Can J Psychiatry 52(4):233–40. DOI:10.1177/070674370705200405.

Lee CH, Giuliana F. 2019. The role of inflammation in depression and
fatigue. *Front Immunol* 10:1696. DOI:10.3389/fimmu.2019.01696.

Lee J. 2020. A neuropsychological exploration of Zoom fatigue.
Psych Times, Nov. 17, 2020. https://www.psychiatrictimes.com/view
/psychological-exploration-zoom-fatigue.

Levine GN, Cohen BE, Commodore-Mensah Y, et al. 2021. Psychological
health, well-being and the mind-heart-body connection. *Circulation*
143:e763–e783. DOI:10.1161/CIR.0000000000000947.

Loades ME, Chatburn E, Higson-Sweeney N, et al. 2020. Rapid systematic
review: The impact of social isolation and loneliness on the mental
health of children and adolescents in the context of COVID-19. *J Am
Acad Child Adolesc Psychiatry* 59(11):1218–39.

McGinty EE, Presskreischer R, Anderson KE, et al. 2020a. Psychological
distress and COVID-19-related stressors reported in a longitudinal
cohort of US adults in April and July 2020. *JAMA* 324(24):2555–57.
DOI:10.1001/jama.2020.21231.

McGinty EE, Presskreischer R, Han H, Barry CL. 2020b. Psychological
distress and loneliness reported by US adults in 2018 and April 2020.
JAMA 324(1):93–94. DOI:10.1001/jama.2020.9740.

Mental wellness for health professionals: COVID-19 and response and
strategies for the future. 2020. Harvard Medical School: Continuing
Education Program. Livestream on Oct. 13–15 and 20–22, 2020.

Murthy VH. 2020. *Together: The Healing Power of Human Connection in
a Sometimes Lonely World*. New York: HarperCollins.

NAMI. 2021. The Impact of COVID-19 on the Mental Health of Young
Adults. NAMI Massachusetts Annual Convention 2021, Healing and
Thriving: Our Path Forward Together. Livestream on November 6,
2021.

Nobel, J. 2021. The COVID-19 pandemic: Now is the time for primary
care to address loneliness. The Foundation for Art and Healing:

The UnLonely Project. Accessed February 2021. https://www
.artandhealing.org/covid-19-now-is-the-time-for-primary-care-to
-address-loneliness/.

O'Connor RC, Wetherall K, Cleare S, et al. 2020. Mental health and
well-being during the COVID-19 pandemic: Longitudinal analyses
of adults in the UK COVID-19 Mental Health and Wellbeing Study.
Br J Psychiatry, Oct. 21, 2020, 1–8. Online. DOI:10.1192/bjp.2020.212.

Parker K, Minkin R, Bennett J. 2020. Economic fallout from COVID-19
continues to hit lower-income Americans the hardest. Pew Research
Center, Sept. 24, 2020. https://www.pewsocialtrends.org/2020/09/24
/economic-fallout-from-covid-19-continues-to-hit-lower-income
-americans-the-hardest/#one-third-of-adults-who-said-they-were-laid
-off-because-of-the-coronavirus-outbreak-are-back-in-their-old-jobs.

Patel SY, Mehrotra A, Huskamp HA, et al. 2020. Trends in outpatient
care delivery and telemedicine during the COVID-19 pandemic in
the US. *JAMA Int Med*, November 16, 2020. Online. DOI:10.1001
/jamainternmed.2020.5928.

Pietrabissa G, Simpson S. 2020. Psychological consequences of social isolation during COVID-19 outbreak. *Front Psychol* 11:2201. DOI:10.3389
/fpsyg.2020.02201.

Rokach A. 2018. The effect of gender and culture on loneliness: A mini
review. *Emerging Science Journ* 2(2):59–64.

Rothbard NP. 2020. Building work-life boundaries in the WFH era.
Harvard Bus Rev, July 15, 2020. https://hbr.org/2020/07/building
-work-life-boundaries-in-the-wfh-era.

Smith BJ, Lim MH. 2020. How the COVID-19 pandemic is focusing attention on loneliness and social isolation. *Public Health Res Pract* 30(2):
e3022008. https://doi.org/10.17061/phrp3022008.

Smith BM, Twohy AJ, Smith GS. 2020. Psychological inflexibility and
intolerance of uncertainty moderate the relationship between social
isolation and mental health outcomes during COVID-19. *J Contextual
Behav Sci* 18:162–74. https://doi.org/10.1016/j.jcbs.2020.09.005.

Southwick SM, Charney DS. 2012. *Resilience: The Science of Mastering
Life's Greatest Challenges*. Cambridge: Cambridge University Press.

Sweet J. 2021. The loneliness pandemic: The psychology and social costs
of isolation in everyday life. *Harvard Magazine*, Jan.–Feb. 2021, 31–36.

Vahratian A, Blumberg SJ, Terlizzi EP, Schiller JS. 2021. Symptoms of
anxiety or depressive disorder and use of mental health care
among adults during the COVID-19 pandemic—United States,

August 2020–February 2021. *MMWR Morb Mortal Wkly Rep*, March 26, 2021. http://dx.doi.org/10.15585/mmwr.mm7013e2.

Valtora NK, Kanaan M, ilbody S, et al. 2016. Loneliness and social isolation as risk factors for coronary heart disease and stroke: Systematic review and meta-analysis of longitudinal observational studies. *Heart* 102:1009–16. DOI:10.1136/heartjnl-2015-308790.

Van Dyke ME, Rogers TM, Pevzner E, et al. 2020. Trends in count-level COVID-19 incidence in counties with and without a mask mandate— Kansas, June 1–August 23, 2020. *MMWR Morb Mortal Wkly Rep* 6(47): 1777–81. https://www.cdc.gov/mmwr/volumes/69/wr/pdfs/mm6947e2 -H.pdf.

Wang J, Mann F, Lloyd-Evans B, et al. 2018. Associations between loneliness and perceived social support and outcomes of mental health problems: A systematic review. *BMC Psychiatry* 18:156. https://doi.org/10.1186/s12888-018-1736-5.

World Health Organization (WHO). 2020. Coronavirus disease (COVID-19). October 2020. https://www.who.int/emergencies/diseases/novel -coronavirus-2019/.

Chapter 2. Stress and Coping Skills

Angold A, Costello EJ, Farmer EMZ, et al. 1999. Impaired but undiagnosed. *J Am Acad Child Adolesc Psychiatry* 38(2):129–37.

Benson H. 2001. *The Relaxation Response*. New York: HarperCollins.

Brooks HL, Rushton K, Lovell K et al. 2018. The power of support from companion animals for people living with mental health problems: A systematic review and narrative synthesis of the evidence. *BMC Psychiatry* 18(31). Online. DOI:10.1186/s12888-018-1613-2.

Centers for Disease Control and Prevention. 2021. Healthy pets, healthy people: How to stay healthy around pets. Last reviewed Sept. 15, 2021. https://www.cdc.gov/healthypets/health-benefits/index.html.

Cherniack EP, Cherniack AR. 2014. The benefit of pets and animal-assisted therapy to the health of older individuals. *Curr Geront and Geriatrics Res* 2014:623203. http://dx.doi.org/10.1155/2014/623203.

Dowling D. 2020. A way forward for working parents. *Harvard Bus Rev*, Nov. 11, 2020. https://hbr.org/2020/11/a-way-forward-for-working -parents.

Fosslein L, West Duffy M. 2020. How to combat Zoom fatigue. *Harvard Bus Rev*, April 29, 2020. https://hbr.org/2020/04/how-to-combat-zoom -fatigue.

Koh C. Why the parental pandemic wall feels so bad right now, and what you can do about it. *Washington Post,* March 8, 2021.

Lee AM, Wong, JGWS, McAloan GM, et al. 2007. Stress and psychological distress among SARS survivors 1 year after the outbreak. *Can J Psychiatry* 52(4):233–40. DOI:10.1177/070674370705200405.

Loades ME, Chatburn E, Higson-Sweeney N, et al. 2020. Rapid systematic review: The impact of social isolation and loneliness on the mental health of children and adolescents in the context of COVID-19. *J Am Acad Child Adolec Psychiatry* 59(11):1218–39.

McConnell AR, Brown CM, Shoda TM. 2011. Friends with benefits: On the positive consequences of pet ownership. *J Personality and Soc Psychology* 101(6):1239–52.

McGinty EE, Presskreischer R, Anderson KE, et al. 2020. Psychological distress and COVID-19-related stressors reported in a longitudinal cohort of US adults in April and July 2020. *JAMA* 324(24):2555–57. DOI:10.1001/jama.2020.21231.

Reynolds G. N.d. The Scientific 7 Minute Workout. *New York Times* Well Workouts, n.d. https://www.nytimes.com/interactive/projects/well/workouts/.

Rothbard NP. 2020. Building work-life boundaries in the WFH era. *Harvard Bus Rev,* July 15, 2020. https://hbr.org/2020/07/building-work-life-boundaries-in-the-wfh-era.

Mindfulness

Kabat-Zinn J. 1994. *Wherever You Go, There You Are.* New York: Hyperion.

Linehan MM. 1993. *Skills Training Manual for Treating Borderline Personality Disorder.* New York: Guilford Press.

Lombardi L, ed. 2017. *Mindfulness: The New Science of Health and Happiness.* New York: Time Special Edition.

Segal ZV, Williams JMG, and Teasdale JD. *Mindfulness-Based Cognitive Therapy for Depression.* New York: Guilford Press, 2002.

Chapter 3. Facing Our Fears

Centers for Disease Control and Prevention (CDC). 2021. COVID-19: Understanding mRNA COVID-19 vaccines. Updated November 3, 2021. https://www.cdc.gov/coronavirus/2019-ncov/vaccines/different-vaccines/mRNA.html.

Fitzpatrick KM, Drawve G, Harris C. 2020. Facing new fears during the COVID-19 pandemic: The state of America's mental health. *J Anxiety Disord* 75:102291. DOI:10.1016/j.janxdis.2020.102291.

Mertens G, Gerritsen L, Duijndam S, et al. 2020. Fear of the coronavirus (COVID-19): Predictors in an online study conducted in March 2020. *J Anxiety Disord* 74:102258. https://doi.org/10.1016/j.janxdis.2020 .102258.

Patel SY, Mehrotra A, Huskamp HA, et al. 2020. Trends in outpatient care delivery and telemedicine during the COVID-19 pandemic in the US. *JAMA Int Med*, November 16, 2020. Online. DOI:10.1001 /jamainternmed.2020.5928.

Southwick SM, Charney DS. 2012. *Resilience: The Science of Mastering Life's Greatest Challenges*. Cambridge: Cambridge University Press.

World Health Organization (WHO). 2020. Pulse survey on continuity of essential health services during the COVID-19 pandemic. August 27, 2020. https://www.who.int/publications/i/item/WHO-2019-nCoV-EHS _continuity-survey-2020.1.

Chapter 4. Fatigue and Burnout

Fatigue

Arnold LM. 2008. Understanding fatigue in major depressive disorder and other medical disorders. *Psychosomatics* 49(3):185–90.

Baldwin DS, Papakostas GI. 2006. Symptoms of fatigue and sleepiness in major depressive disorder. *J Clin Psych* 67(suppl 6):9–15.

Nierenberg AA, Husain MM, Trivedi MH, et al. 2010. Residual symptoms after remission of major depressive disorder with citalopram and risk of relapse: A STAR*D report. *Psychol Med* 40(1):41–50.

Nierenberg AA, Keefe BR, Leslie VC, et al. 1999. Residual symptoms in depressed patients who respond acutely to fluoxetine. *J Clin Psych* 60(4):221–25.

Burnout

Abramson A. 2021. The impact of parental burnout: What psychological research suggests how to recognize and overcome it. *Am Psychological Assoc*, October 1, 2021. https://www.apa.org/monitor/2021/10/cover -parental-burnout.

Griffith AK. 2020. Parental burnout and child maltreatment during the COVID-19 pandemic. *J Fam Violence*, Jun 23:1–7. DOI: 10.1007/s10896 -020-00172-2.

HBR. 2021. *HBR Guide to Beating Burnout*. Boston: Harvard Business Review Press.

McBride L. 2021. By now, burnout is a given. *Atlantic*, June 30, 2021. https://www.theatlantic.com/ideas/archive/2021/06/burnout-medical-condition-pandemic/619321/.

Maslach C, Leiter MP. 2005. Reversing burnout: How to rekindle your passion for your work. *Stanford Soc Innov Rev*, Winter 2005. https://ssir.org/articles/entry/reversing_burnout#.

Maslach C, Leiter MP. 2016. Understanding the burnout experience: Recent research and its implications for psychiatry. *World Psychiatry* 15(2):103–11.

Mikolajczak M, Brianda ME, Avalosse H, Roskam I. 2018. Consequences of parental burnout: Its specific effect on child neglect and violence. *Child Abuse and Neglect* 80:134–45. DOI:10.1016/j.chiabu.2018.03.025.

Rionda IS, Cortés-Garcia L, de la Villa Moral Jiménez M. 2021. The role of burnout in the association between work-related factors and perceived errors in clinical practice among Spanish residents. *Int J Environ Res Public Health* 18(9):4931.

Valcour M. 2016. Beating burnout. *Harvard Bus Rev*, November 2016. https://hbr.org/2016/11/beating-burnout.

World Health Organization (WHO). 2019. Burn-out an occupational phenomenon: International classification of diseases. *WHO: Departmental News*, May 28, 2019. https://www.who.int/news/item/28-05-2019-burn-out-an-occupational-phenomenon-international-classification-of-diseases.

Chapter 5. The Ability to Grieve

Berinato S. 2020. That discomfort you're feeling is grief. *Harvard Bus Rev*, March 23, 2020. https://hbr.org/2020/03/that-discomfort-youre-feeling-is-grief.

Bryant RA, Kenny L, Joscelyne A, et al. 2014. Treating prolonged grief disorder: A randomized clinical trial. *JAMA Psychiatry* 71(12):1332–39. DOI:10.1001/jamapsychiatry.2014.1600.

Carr D, Boerner K, Moorman S. 2020. Bereavement in the time of coronavirus: Unprecedented challenges demand novel interventions. *J Aging Soc Policy* 32(4–5):425–31. DOI:10.1080/08959420.2020.1764320.

Centers for Disease Control and Prevention. 2020. Grief and loss. June 11, 2020. https://www.cdc.gov/coronavirus/2019-ncov/daily-life-coping/stress-coping/grief-loss.html.

Columbia Center for Complicated Grief. 2021. Overview. Accessed March 2021. https://complicatedgrief.columbia.edu/professionals/complicated -grief-professionals/overview/.

Goveas JS, Shear K. 2020. Grief and the COVID-19 pandemic in older adults. *Am J Geriatr Psychiatry* 28(10):1119–25.

Killikelly C, Maercker A. 2018. Prolonged grief disorder for ICD-11: The primacy of clinical utility and international applicability. *Europ J Psychotraumatology* 8:1476441. https://doi.org/10.1080 /20008198.2018.1476441.

Koh C. 2021. Why the parental pandemic wall feels so bad right now, and what you can do about it. *Washington Post*, March 8, 2021.

Kübler-Ross E. (1969) 2014. *On Death and Dying*. New York: Simon & Schuster.

Kübler-Ross E, Kessler D. 2014. *On Grief and Grieving: Finding the Meaning of Grief through the Five Stages of Loss*. New York: Scribner.

Maercker A, Lalor J. 2012. Diagnostic and clinical considerations in prolonged grief disorder. *Dialogues Clin Neurosci* 14(2):167–76.

Zhai Y, Du X. 2020. Loss and grief amidst COVID-19: A path to adaptation and resilience. *Brain, Behavior and Immunity* 87:80–81. https:// doi.org/10.1016/j.bbi.2020.04.053.

Chapter 6. Isolation and Mental Health

American Psychiatric Association (APA). 2013. *Diagnostic and Statistical Manual of Mental Disorders (DSM-5)*. 5th ed. Arlington, VA: American Psychiatric Association.

Angold A, Costello EJ, Farmer EMZ, et al. 1999. Impaired but undiagnosed. *J Am Acad Child Adolesc Psychiatry* 38(2):129–37.

Anxiety

Anxiety and Depression Association of America. 2021. COVID-19 anxiety. ADAA, last updated Sept. 28, 2021. https://adaa.org/finding-help /coronavirus-anxiety-helpful-resources.

Fava M, Alpert JE, Carmin CN, et al. 2004. Clinical correlates and symptom patterns of anxious depression among patients with major depressive disorder in STAR*D. *Psychol Med* 34:1299–308.

Melton TH, Croarkin PE, Strawn JR, McClintock SM. 2016. Comorbid anxiety and depressive symptoms in children and adolescents: A systematic review and analysis. *J Psychiatr Pract* 22(2):84–98.

Regier DA, Rae DS, Narrow WE, Kaelber CT, Schatzberg AF. 1998. Prevalence of anxiety disorders and their comorbidity with mood and addictive disorders. *Br J Psychiatry Suppl* 34:24–28.

Stein MB, Sareen J. 2015. Generalized anxiety disorder. *N Engl J Med* 373(21):2059–68.

Van Ameringen M. 2021. Comorbid anxiety and depression in adults: Epidemiology, clinical manifestations, and diagnosis. *UpToDate*, last updated April 13, 2021. https://www.uptodate.com/contents /comorbid-anxiety-and-depression-in-adults-epidemiology-clinical -manifestations-and-diagnosis.

Depression

aan het Rot M, Collins KA, Murrough JW, et al. 2010. Safety and efficacy of repeated-dose intravenous ketamine for treatment-resistant depression. *Biol Psychiatry* 67(2):139–45.

Al-Harbi KS. 2012. Treatment resistant depression: Therapeutic trends, challenges, and future directions. *Patient Prefer Adherence* 6:369–88.

Altemus M. 2017. Neuroendocrine networks and functionality. *Psychiatr Clin North Am* 40(2):189–200.

Andrade AC. 2015. Intranasal drug delivery in neuropsychiatry: Focus on intranasal ketamine for refractory depression. *J Clin Psychiatry* 76(5):e628–31.

Beck AT, Alford BA. 2009. *Depression: Causes and Treatment*. Philadelphia: University of Pennsylvania Press.

Berlim MT, Turecki G. 2007. Definition, assessment, and staging of treatment-resistant refractory major depression: A review of current concepts and methods. *Can J Psychiatry* 52(1):46–54.

Bilello JA. 2016. Seeking an objective diagnosis of depression. *Biomark Med* 10(8):861–75.

Bromberger JT, Schott L, Kravitz HM, Joffe H. 2015. Risk factors for major depression during midlife among a community sample of women with and without prior major depression: Are they the same or different? *Psychol Med* 45(8):1653–64.

Conway CR, George MS, Sackeim HS. 2017. Toward an evidence-based, operational definition of treatment-resistant depression: When enough is enough. *JAMA Psychiatry* 74(1):9–10.

Cuijpers P, Weitz E, Karyotaki E, et al. 2015. The effects of psychological treatment of maternal depression on children and parental functioning: A meta-analysis. *Eur Child Adolesc Psychiatry*. 24(2):237–45. DOI:10.1007/s00787-014-0660-6.

Fava M, Alpert JE, Carmin CN, et al. 2004. Clinical correlates and symptom patterns of anxious depression among patients with major depressive disorder in STAR*D. *Psychol Med* 34(7):1299–308.

Goodman SH, Garber J. 2017. Evidence-based interventions for depressed mothers and their young children. *Child Dev* 88(2):368–77. DOI:10.1111/cdev.12732.

Hyde CL, Nagle MW, Tian C, et al. 2016. Identification of 15 genetic loci associated with risk of major depression in individuals of European descent. *Nat Genet* 48(9):1031–36. DOI:10.1038/ng.3623.

MacKinnon DF. 2016. *Still Down: What to Do When Antidepressants Fail.* Baltimore, MD: Johns Hopkins University Press.

Marcus SAM, Young EA, Kerber KB, et al. 2005. Gender differences in depression: Findings from the STAR*D study. *J Affect Disord* 87(2–3): 141–50.

Martin LA, Neighbors HW, Griffith DM. 2013. The experience of symptoms of depression in men vs women: Analysis of the National Comorbidity Survey replication. *JAMA Psychiatry* 70(10):1100–106.

McAllister-Williams RH, Arango C, Blier P, et al. 2020. The identification, assessment and management of difficult-to-treat depression: An international consensus statement. *J Affect Dis* 267:264–82. https://doi.org/10.1016/j.jad.2020.02.023.

Murrough JW, Iosifescu DV, Chang LC, et al. 2013. Antidepressant efficacy of ketamine in treatment-resistant major depression: A two-site randomized controlled trial. *Am J Psychiatry* 170(10):1134–42.

Noonan SJ. 2018. *Take Control of Your Depression: Strategies to Help You Feel Better Now.* Baltimore, MD: Johns Hopkins University Press.

Rush AJ, Aaronson ST, Demyttenaere K. 2019. Difficult-to-treat depression: A clinical and research roadmap for when remission is elusive. *Australian and New Zealand J Psychiatry* 53(2):109–18. DOI:10.1177/0004867418808585.

Rush AJ, Trivedi MH, Wisniewski SR, et al. 2006. Acute and longer-term outcomes in depressed outpatients requiring one or several treatment steps: A STAR*D Report. *Am J Psychiatry* 163(11):1905–17.

Saveanu RV, Nemeroff CB. 2012. Etiology of depression: Genetic and environmental factors. *Psychiatr Clin North Am* 35(1):51–71.

Sullivan PF, Neale MC, Kendler KS. 2000. Genetic epidemiology of major depression: Review and meta-analysis. *Am J Psychiatry* 157(10):1552–62.

Trevino K, McClintock SM, McDonald Fisher N, et al. 2014. Defining treatment-resistant depression: A comprehensive review of the literature. *Ann Clin Psychiatry* 26(3):222–32.

Trivedi MH, Rush AJ, Wisniewski SR, et al. 2006. Evaluation of outcomes with citalopram for depression using measurement-based care in STAR*D: Implication for clinical practice. *Am J Psychiatry* 163(1):28–40.

Yeung A, Feldman G, Fava M. 2010. *Self-Management of Depression: A Manual for Mental Health and Primary Care Professionals.* Cambridge: Cambridge University Press.

PTSD

Department of Veterans Affairs (VA) and Department of Defense (DOD). 2017. VA/DOD clinical practice guideline for the management of posttraumatic stress disorder and acute stress disorder. Version 3.0— 2017. https://www.healthquality.va.gov/guidelines/MH/ptsd/VADOD PTSDCPGFinal082917.pdf.

Hawryluck L, Gold WL, Robinson S, et al. 2004. SARS control and psychological effects of quarantine, Toronto, Canada. *Emerg Infect Dis* 10:1206–12.

Janiri D, Carfi A, Kotzalidid GD, et al. 2021. Posttraumatic stress disorder in patients after severe COVID-19 infection. *JAMA Psychiatry* 78(5): 567 69. DOI:10.1001/jamapsychiatry.20210109.

National Center for PTSD. 2021. PTSD Basics. US Department of Veterans Affairs, last updated June 15, 2021. https://www.ptsd.va.gov/understand /what/ptsd_basics.asp.

Rothbaum BO, Rauch SAM. 2020. *PTSD: What Everyone Needs to Know.* Oxford: Oxford University Press.

Yehuda R. 2002. Post-traumatic stress disorder. *N Engl J Med* 346(2);108–14.

Post-traumatic Growth

Tedeschi RG, Calhoun LG. 1996. The posttraumatic growth inventory: Measuring the positive legacy of trauma. *J Traum Stress* 9(3):455–71.

Chapter 7. Suicidal Thoughts or Impulses

American Foundation for Suicide Prevention (AFSP). 2021a. Risk factors, protective factors, and warning signs. Accessed January 2021. https:// afsp.org/risk-factors-and-warning-signs.

American Foundation for Suicide Prevention (AFSP). 2021b. Suicide facts and figures: United States 2020. Accessed January 2021. https:// www.datocms-assets.com/12810/1587128056-usfactsfiguresflyer-2.pdf.

Beyer JL, Weisler RH. 2016. Suicide behaviors in bipolar disorder: A review and update for the clinician. *Psychiatr Clin North Am* 39(1):111–23.

Centers for Disease Control and Prevention (CDC). 2021a. Risk and protective factors. Last reviewed May 13, 2021. https://www.cdc.gov/suicide/factors/index.html.

Centers for Disease Control and Prevention (CDC). 2021b. Suicide and self-harm injury. Last reviewed Sept. 13, 2021. https://www.cdc.gov/nchs/fastats/suicide.htm.

Czeisler MÉ, Lane RI, Petrosky E, et al. 2020. Mental health, substance use, and suicidal ideation during the COVID-19 pandemic—United States, June 24–30, 2020. *MMWR Morb Mortal Wkly Rep* 69:1049–57. http://dx.doi.org/10.15585/mmwr.mm6932a1.

Dazzi T, Gribble R, Wessely S, et al. 2014. Does asking about suicide and related behaviours induce suicidal ideation? What is the evidence? *Psychol Med* 44(16):3361–63.

Fazel S, Runeson B. 2020. Suicide. *N Engl J Med* 382:266–74.

Lardier DT Jr., Barrios VR, Garcia-Reid P, Reid RJ. 2016. Suicidal ideation among suburban adolescents: The influence of school bullying and other mediating risk factors. *J Child Adolesc Ment Health* 28(3):213–31.

McClatchey K, Murray J, Rowat A, Chouliara Z. 2017. Risk factors for suicide and suicidal behavior relevant to emergency health care settings: A systematic review of post-2007 reviews. *Suicide Life Threat Behav* 47(6):729–45.

Miron O, Yu K, Wilf-Miron R, Kohane IS. 2019. Suicide rates among adolescents and young adults in the United States, 2000–2017. *JAMA* 321(23):2362–64. DOI:10.1001/jama.2019.5054.

Olson R. 2014. Why do people kill themselves? Centre for Suicide Prevention. https://www.suicideinfo.ca/resource/suicidetheories/.

Steinhauer JVA. 2019. Officials, and the nation, battle an unrelenting tide of veteran suicides. *New York Times*, April 14, 2019.

Stone DM, Simon TR, Fowler, KA, et al. 2018. Vital signs: Trends in state suicide rates—United States, 1999–2016, and circumstances contributing to suicide—27 states, 2015. *MMWR Morb Mortal Wkly Rep* 67(22):617–24. https://www.cdc.gov/mmwr/volumes/67/wr/pdfs/mm6722a1-H.pdf.

Turecki G, Brent DA. 2016. Suicide and suicidal behaviour. *Lancet* 387(10024):1227–39.

Chapter 8. Substance Abuse and Addictions

Blanco C, Alegria AA, Liu SM, et al. 2012. Differences among major depressive disorder with and without co-occurring substance use disorders and substance-induced depressive disorder: Results from the National Epidemiologic Survey on Alcohol and Related Conditions. *J Clin Psychiatry* 73(6):865–73.

DiForti M, Quattrone D, Freeman TP, et al. 2019. The contribution of cannabis use to variation in the incidence of psychotic disorder across Europe (EU-GEI): A multicenter case-control study. *Lancet Psychiatry* 6(5):427–36. http://doi.org/10.1016/S2215-0366(19)30048-3.

Gobbi G, Atkin T, Zytynski T, et al. 2019. Association of cannabis use in adolescence and risk of depression, anxiety, and suicidality in young adulthood: A systematic review and meta-analysis. *JAMA Psychiatry* 76(4):426–34.

Kessler RC. 2004. The epidemiology of dual diagnosis. *Biol Psychiatry* 56:730–37.

Mark TL. 2003. The costs of treating persons with depression and alcoholism compared with depression alone. *Psych Serv* 54(8):1095–97.

NAMI. 2015. Dual diagnosis. Updated March 2015. https://www.nami.org/NAMI/media/NAMI-Media/Images/FactSheets/Dual-Diagnosis-FS.pdf.

NAMI. 2020. Substance use disorders. Last reviewed May 2020. https://www.nami.org/About-Mental-Illness/Common-with-Mental-Illness/Substance-Use-Disorders.

SAMHSA. Behavioral health trends in the United States: Results from the 2014 National Survey on Drug Use and Health. Sept. 2015. https://www.samhsa.gov/data/sites/default/files/NSDUH-FRR1-2014/NSDUH-FRR1-2014.pdf.

Schrier LA, Harris SK, Kurland M, Knight JR. 2003. Substance use problems and associated psychiatric symptoms among adolescents in primary care. *Pediatrics* 111(6 Pt 1):e699–705.

Chapter 9. Understanding the Basics of Mental Health

Sleep
American Academy of Sleep Medicine. 2020. Healthy sleep habits. Updated August 2020. http://sleepeducation.org/essentials-in-sleep/healthy-sleep-habits.

Asarnow LD, Manber R. 2019. Cognitive behavioral therapy for insomnia in depression. *Sleep Med Clin* 14(2):177–84.

National Institute of Neurologic Disorders and Stroke. 2019. Brain basics: Understanding sleep. NIH Publication No. 17-3440c. Last modified Aug. 13, 2019. https://www.ninds.nih.gov/Disorders/Patient-Caregiver -Education/Understanding-Sleep.

Sleep Foundation. 2020. Sleep hygiene. Updated Aug. 14, 2020. https:// www.sleepfoundation.org/sleep-hygiene.

Tsuno N, Besset S, Ritchie K. 2005. Sleep and depression. *J Clin Psychiatry* 66(10):1254–69.

Winkelman JW. 2020. How to identify and fix sleep problems: Better sleep, better mental health. *JAMA Psychiatry* 77(1):99–100. DOI:10.100 /jamapsychiatry.2019.3832.

Nutrition

Berk M, Jacka FN. 2019. Diet and depression—from confirmation to implementation. *JAMA* 321(9):842–43.

Bodnar LM, Wisner KL. 2005. Nutrition and depression: Implications for improving mental health among childbearing-aged women. *Biol Psychiatry* 58(9):679–85.

Diet and depression. 2019. *Tufts University Diet and Nutrition Letter* 36(11):6–7.

Firth J, Marx W, Dash S, et al. 2019. The effects of dietary improvement on symptoms of depression and anxiety: A meta-analysis of randomized controlled trials. *Psychosom Med* 81(3):264–80. DOI:10.1097 /PSY.0000000000000673.

Jacka FN, O'Neil A, Opie R, et al. 2017. A randomized controlled trial of dietary improvement for adults with major depression (the "SMILES" trial). *BMC Med* 15(1):23. DOI:10.1186/s12916-017-0791-y.

Jacka FN, Pasco JA, Mykletun A, et al. 2010. Association of Western and traditional diets with depression and anxiety in women. *Am J Psychiatry* 167(3):305–11.

Khalid S, Williams CM, Reynolds SA. 2016. Is there an association between diet and depression in children and adolescents? A systematic review. *Br J Nutr* 116(12):2097–108.

Ma J, Rosas LG, Lv N, et al. 2019. Effect of integrated behavioral weight loss treatment and problem-solving therapy on body mass index and depressive symptoms among patients with obesity and depression: The RAINBOW randomized clinical trial. *JAMA* 321(9):869–79. DOI:10.1001/jama20190557.

Mayo Clinic. 2021. Mediterranean diet for hearth health. Mayo Clinic, July 23, 2021. http://www.mayoclinic.org/healthy-lifestyle/nutrition -and-healthy-eating/in-depth/mediterranean-diet/art-20047801.

Sanchez-Villegas A, Delgado-Rodriguez M, Schlatter AA, et al. 2009. Association of the Mediterranean dietary pattern with the incidence of depression: The Seguimiento Universidad de Navarra/University of Navarro follow up. *Arch Gen Psychiatry* 66(10):1090–98.

US Department of Agriculture (USDA). 2021. My plate. Accessed April 2021. https://www.myplate.gov/.

US Department of Agriculture and US Department of Health and Human Services. 2020. *Dietary Guidelines for Americans, 2020–2025*. 9th ed. Washington, DC: Government Printing Office. https://www.dietary guidelines.gov/sites/default/files/2020-12/Dietary_Guidelines_for _Americans_2020-2025.pdf.

Physical Exercise

Carter T, Morres ID, Meade O, Callaghan P. 2016. The effect of exercise on depressive symptoms in adolescents: A systematic review and meta-analysis. *J Am Acad Child Adolesc Psychiatry* 55(7):580–90.

Choi KW, Chen CY, Stein MB, et al. 2019. Assessment of bidirectional relationships between physical activity and depression among adults: A 2-sample Mendelian randomization study. *JAMA Psychiatry* 76(4): 399–408.

Cooney GM, Dwan K, Greig CA, et al. 2013. Exercise for depression. *Cochrane Database Syst Rev* 9(9):CD004366.

Cooney G, Dwan K, Mead G. 2014. Exercise for depression. *JAMA* 311(23): 2432–33.

Cotman CW, Berchtold NC, Christie LA. 2007. Exercise builds brain health: Key roles of growth factor cascades and inflammation. *Trends Neurosci* 30(9):464–72.

Dunn AL, Trivedi MH, Kampert JB, Clark CG, Chambliss HO. 2005. Exercise treatment for depression: Efficacy and dose response. *Am J Prev Med* 28(1):1–8.

Harvey SB, Øverland S, Hatch SL, Wessely S, Mykletun A, Hotopf M. 2018. Exercise and the prevention of depression: Results of the HUNT cohort study. *Am J Psychiatry* 175(1):28–36.

Hoare E, Milton K, Foster C, Allender S. 2016. The associations between sedentary behaviour and mental health among adolescents: A systematic review. *Int J Behav Nutr Phys Act* 13(1):108.

McMahon EM, Corcoran P, O'Regan G, et al. 2017. Physical activity in European adolescents and associations with anxiety, depression and well-being. *Eur Child Adolesc Psychiatry* 26(1):111–22.

Melo MCA, Daher EDF, Albuquerque SGC, de Bruin VMS. 2016. Exercise in bipolar patients: A systematic review. *J Affect Disord* 198:32–38.

Morres ID, Hatzigeorgiadis A, Stathi A, et al. 2019. Aerobic exercise for adult patients with major depressive disorder in mental health services: A systematic review and meta-analysis. *Depress Anxiety* 36(1):39–53.

Murri MB, Ekkekakis P, Menchetti M, et al. 2018. Physical exercise for late-life depression: Effects on symptom dimensions and time course. *J Affect Disord* 230:65–70.

Piercy KL, Troiano RP, Ballard RM, et al. 2018. The physical activity guidelines for Americans. *JAMA* 320(19):2020–28.

Rethorst CD, Trivedi MH. 2013. Evidence-based recommendations for the prescription of exercise for major depressive disorder. *J Psychiatr Pract* 19(3):204–12.

Rethorst CD, Wipfli BM, Landers DM. 2009. The antidepressant effect of exercise: A meta-analysis of randomized trials. *Sports Med.* 39(6): 491–511.

Schuch FB, Vancampfort D, Richards J, Rosenbaum S, Ward PB, Stubbs B. 2016. Exercise as a treatment for depression: A meta-analysis adjusting for publication bias. *J Psychiatr Res* 77:42–51.

Trivedi MH, Greer TL, Grannemann BD, et al. 2006. Exercise as an augmentation strategy for treatment of major depression. *J Psychiatr Pract* 12(4):205–13.

US Department of Health and Human Services (HHS). 2018. *Physical Activity Guidelines for Americans.* 2nd ed. Washington, DC: HHS. https://health.gov/paguidelines/second-edition/pdf/Physical_Activity _Guidelines_2nd_edition.pdf.

Vancampfort D, Stubbs B, Firth J, Van Damme T, Koyanagi A. 2018. Sedentary behavior and depressive symptoms among 67,077 adolescents aged 12–15 years from 30 low- and middle-income countries. *Int J Behav Nutr Phys Act* 15(1):73.

Yang L, Cao C, Kantor ED, et al. 2019. Trends in sedentary behavior among the US population, 2001–2016. *JAMA* 321(16):1587–97.

Chapter 10. Finding Effective Professional Mental Health Care

Bower AJ, Gilbody S, Lovell K. et al. 2012. Collaborative care for depression and anxiety problems. *Cochrane Database Sys Rev* 10:2.

Carlo AD, Barnett BS, Unutzer J. 2020. Harnessing collaborative care to meet mental health demands in the era of COVID-19. *JAMA Psychiatry* 78(4):355–56. DOI:10.1001/jamapsychiatry.2020.3216.

Fortney JC, Pyne JM, Kimbrell TA, et al. 2015. Telemedicine-based collaborative care for posttraumatic stress disorder: A randomized clinical trial. *JAMA Psychiatry* 72(1):58–67. DOI:10.1001/jamapsychiatry .2014.1575.

Haselden M, Brister T, Robinson S, Covell N, Pauselli L, Dixon L. 2019. Effectiveness of the NAMI Homefront program for military and veteran families: In-person and online benefits. *Psychiatr Serv* 70(10): 935–39. https://doi.org/10.1176/appi.ps.201800573.

Highet N, Thompson M, McNair B. 2005. Identifying depression in a family member: The carers' experience. *J Affect Disord* 87:25–33.

Noonan SJ. 2013. *Managing Your Depression: What You Can Do to Feel Better*. Baltimore, MD: Johns Hopkins University Press.

Patel SY, Mehrotra A, Huskamp HA, et al. 2020. Trends in outpatient care delivery and telemedicine during the Covid-19 pandemic in the US. *JAMA Int Med* 181(3):388–91. Online. DOI:10.1001/jamainternmed .2020.5928.

Rauch SAM, Simon N, Rothbaum B. 2020. Phased approach for supporting the mental health of healthcare workers and others affected by the COVID-19 pandemic (PAC). ADAA. May 4, 2020. https://adaa.org /sites/default/files/PhasedApproachtoCovid-19.ver1.2.pdf.

Sturmey P. 2009. Behavioral activation is an evidence-based treatment for depression. *Behavior Modification* 33(6):818–29.

Substance Abuse and Mental Health Services Administration (SAMHSA). 2020. *Key Substance Use and Mental Health Indicators in the United States: Results from the 2019 National Survey on Drug Use and Health*. HHS Publication No. PEP20-07-01-001, NSDUH Series H-55. Rockville, MD: Center for Behavioral Health Statistics and Quality, Substance Abuse and Mental Health Services Administration.

Swanson KA, Bastani R, Rubenstein LV, Meridith LS, Ford DE. 2007. Effect of mental health care and shared decision making on patient satisfaction in a community sample of patients with depression. *Med Care Res Rev* 64(4):416–30.

Cultural Differences in Mental Health Care
Carpenter-Song E, Chu Ed, Drake RE, et al. 2010. Ethno-cultural variations in the experience and meaning of mental illness and treatment:
Implications for access and utilization. *Transcult Psychiatry* 47(2):
224–51. DOI:10.1177/1363461510368906.
Gopalkrishnan N. 2018. Cultural diversity and mental health: Considerations for policy and practice. *Front Public Health* 6:179. DOI:10.3389
/fpubh.2018.00179.
Martinez KG. 2019. Influences of cultural differences in the diagnosis
and treatment of anxiety and depression. Anxiety and Depression
Association of America, May 14, 2019. https://adaa.org/learn-from-us
/from-the-experts/blog-posts/consumer/influences-cultural-differences
-diagnosis-and.
Mental Health First Aid (MHFA). 2019. Four ways culture impacts mental
health. MHFA, July 11, 2019. https://www.mentalhealthfirstaid.org
/2019/07/four-ways-culture-impacts-mental-health/.
National Alliance for Mental Illness (NAMI). Identity and cultural dimensions. NAMI. Accessed July 2021. https://www.nami.org/Your-Journey
/Identity-and-Cultural-Dimensions.
US Department of Health and Human Services. 2001. *Mental Health:
Culture, Race, and Ethnicity—A Supplement to Mental Health: A Report
of the Surgeon General.* Rockville, MD: US Department of Health
and Human Services, Substance Abuse and Mental Health Services
Administration, Center for Mental Health Services. https://www.ncbi
.nlm.nih.gov/books/NBK44243/pdf/Bookshelf_NBK44243.pdf.

Chapter 11. Is Talk Therapy Right for Me?

Bryant RA, Kenny L, Joscelyne A, et al. 2014. Treating prolonged grief
disorder: A randomized clinical trial. *JAMA Psychiatry* 71(12):1332–39.
DOI:10.1001/jamapsychoatry.2014.1600.
Department of Veterans Affairs and Department of Defense. 2017.
VA/DOD clinical practice guideline for the management of post-
traumatic stress disorder and acute stress disorder. Version 3.0—
2017. https://www.healthquality.va.gov/guidelines/MH/ptsd/VADO
DPTSDCPGFinal082917.pdf.
Fava GA, Rafanelli C, Grandi S, et al. 1998. Prevention of recurrent
depression with cognitive behavioral therapy: Preliminary findings.
Arch Gen Psychiatry 55(9):816–20.

Harley R, Sprich S, Safran JM, Fava M. 2008. Adaptation of dialectical behavioral therapy skills training group for treatment-resistant depression. *J Nerv Ment Dis* 196(2):136–43.

Harris R. 2011. Embracing your demons: An overview of Acceptance and Commitment Therapy. Psychotherapy.net. https://www.psychotherapy .net/article/Acceptance-and-Commitment-Therapy-ACT#section-the -goal-of-act.

Nierenberg AA, Petersen TJ, Alpert JA. 2003. Prevention of relapse and recurrence in depression: The role of long-term pharmacotherapy and psychotherapy. *J Clin Psychiatry* 64(suppl 15):13–17.

Ostacher MJ, Cifu AS. 2019. Management of posttraumatic stress disorder. *JAMA* 321(2): 200–201.

Patel SY, Mehrotra A, Huskamp HA, et al. 2020. Trends in outpatient care delivery and telemedicine during the Covid-19 pandemic in the US. *JAMA Int Med*, November 16, 2020. Online. DOI:10.1001/jamainternmed .2020.5928.

Petersen TJ. 2006. Enhancing the efficacy of antidepressants with psycho-therapy. *J Psychopharmacol* 20(suppl 3):19–28.

Pierce BS, Perrin PB, Tyler CM, et al. 2021. The COVID-19 telepsychology revolution: A national study of pandemic-based changes in US mental health care delivery. *American Psychologist* 26(1):14–25. https://doi.org /10.1037/amp0000722.

Richards CS, Perri MG, eds. 2010. *Relapse Prevention for Depression.* Washington, DC: American Psychological Association.

Sudak DM. 2012. Cognitive behavioral therapy for depression. *Psychiatr Clin North Am* 35(1):99–110.

Teasdale JD, Segal ZV, Williams JMG, Ridgeway VA, Soulsby JM, Lau MA. 2000. Prevention of relapse/recurrence in major depression by mind-fulness-based cognitive therapy. *J Consul Clin Psychol* 8(4):615–23.

Trivedi MH, Rush AJ, Wisniewski SR, et al. 2006. Evaluation of out-comes with citalopram for depression using measurement-based care in STAR*D: Implication for clinical practice. *Am J Psychiatry* 163(1):28–40.

Yasinski C, Rauch SAM. 2018. A review of recent efforts to improve access to effective psychotherapies. *Focus* (Am Psychiatr Pub) 16(4): 356–62. DOI:10.1176/appi.focus.20180018.

Chapter 12. Building and Maintaining Resilience

American Psychological Association (APA). (2012) 2020. Resilience guide for parents and teachers. APA, Jan. 24, 2012; last updated Aug. 26, 2020. https://www.apa.org/topics/resilience/guide-parents-teachers.

American Psychological Association (APA). 2011. Building your resilience. APA, April 2011. https://www.apaservices.org/practice/good-practice /building-resilience.pdf.

Catalano D, Wilson L, Chan F, Chiu C, Muller VR. 2011. The buffering effect of resilience on depression among individuals with spinal cord injury: A structural equation model. *Rehabil Psychol* 56(3):200–211.

Comas-Diaz L, Luthar SS, Maddi SR, O'Neill HK, Saakvitne KW, Tedeschi RG. 2013. *The Road to Resilience*. Washington, DC: American Psychological Association.

Dunn AL, Trivedi MH, Kampert JB, Clark CG, Chamblis HO. 2005. Exercise treatment for depression: Efficacy and dose response. *Am J Prev Med* 28(1):1–8.

Haeffel GF, Vargas I. 2011. Resilience to depressive symptoms: The buffering effects of enhancing cognitive style and positive life events. *J Behav Ther Exp Psychiatry* 42(1):13–18.

Mak WWS, Ng ISW, Wong CCY. 2011. Resilience: Enhancing well-being through the positive cognitive triad. *J Couns Psychol* 58(4):610–17.

Masten AS. 2001. Ordinary magic: Resilience processes in development. *Am Psychol* 56:227–38.

Mead GE, Morley W, Campbell P, Greig CA, McMurdo M, Lawlor DA. 2009. Exercise for depression. *Cochrane Database of Syst Rev* 3:CD004366.

Newman R. 2002. The road to resilience. *Monitor on Psychology* 33(9):62. https://www.apa.org/monitor/oct02/pp.

Rethorst CD, Trivedi MH. 2013. Evidence-based recommendations for the prescription of exercise for major depressive disorder. *J Psychiatr Pract* 19(3):204–12.

Southwick SM, Charney DS. 2012. *Resilience: The Science of Mastering Life's Greatest Challenges*. Cambridge: Cambridge University Press.

Stein MB, Campbell-Sills L, Gelernter J. 2009. Genetic variation in 5HTTLPR is associated with emotional resilience. *Am J Med Genet B Neuropsychiatr Genet* 150B(7):900–906.

Trivedi MH, Greer TL, Grannemann BD, Chambliss HO, Jordan AN. 2006. Exercise as an augmentation strategy for treatment of major depression. *J Psychiatr Pract* 12(4):205–13.

Vanderhorst RK, McLaren S. 2005. Social relationships as predictors of depression and suicidal ideation in older adults. *Aging Ment Health* 9(6):517–25.

Wingo AP, Wrenn G, Pelletier T, Gutman AR, Bradley B, Ressler KJ. 2010. Moderating effects of resilience on depression in individuals with a history of childhood abuse or trauma exposure. *J Affect Disord* 126(30): 411–14.

Chapter 13. Looking Forward: Reentry Anxiety

American Psychological Association (APA). 2021. Stress in America 2021: Pandemic stress one year on. Stress in America Press Room, March 2021. https://www.apa.org/news/press/releases/stress.

Ducharme J. 2021. How to soothe your "Re-entry Anxiety" as COVID-19 lockdowns lift. *Time*, June 11, 2021. https://time.com/5850143/covid-19 -re-entry-anxiety/.

Mangurian C. 2021. *Re-Entering the Workplace in 2021: A Manager's Guide.* UCSF Cope Well-Being Subgroup. Accessed July 2021. https:// psychiatry.ucsf.edu/sites/psych.ucsf.edu/files/Cope%20Re-Entry%20 Guide%20for%20Managers.pdf.

Pappas S. 2021. Why the pandemic's end spurs anxiety. American Psychological Association, May 4, 2021. https://www.apa.org/topics /covid-19/pandemic-end-anxiety.

Index